Childhood Asthma

Childhood Asthma

A doctor's complete treatment plan

Dr Mike Whiteside

Thorsons
An Imprint of HarperCollins*Publishers*

Thorsons
An Imprint of HarperCollins*Publishers*
77-85 Fulham Palace Road,
Hammersmith, London W6 8JB

Published by Thorsons 1991
10 9 8 7 6 5 4 3 2

A catalogue record for this book is available
from the British Library

ISBN 0 7225 2245 2

Typeset by Harper Phototypesetters Limited
Northampton, England
Printed and bound in Great Britain by
Mackays of Chatham PLC, Chatham, Kent

Contents

Asthma, its Nature and Causes

CHAPTER 1

The Aim of this Book

Asthma is a most unpleasant and frightening condition. The primary aim of this book is to enable both parents and their children to lead a relaxed, normal life without the constant worry and threat of a severe attack. To witness your own child struggling desperately for breath is an extremely distressing experience. As a parent you have a strong protective reflex towards your children and there is always a tremendous desire to ease their suffering; the immediate instinct is to try to breathe for them but of course this is not possible. This anxiety at being unable to ease the shortness of breath soon transmits itself to the child who, instead of being calmly reassured, becomes even more agitated at sensing a mum or dad close to panic. Often the only outcome when this stage is reached is admission to hospital, thus inflicting further stress on both child and parents.

As a father of three children who have all suffered from asthma to varying degrees, I have experienced all these feelings. Even as a doctor it is not always possible to think clearly in the heat of the moment. Five years ago I therefore decided to create a plan of action which would deal with virtually every situation involving an asthmatic child. At that time approximately one child on my patient list was being admitted to hospital per week, but by perfecting this system of management I have cut admissions to virtually nil. In fact no children registered on my list have been sent into hospital in the past year.

Asthma is a serious and potentially dangerous condition which can come on with alarming speed. There are two thousand deaths from asthma every year in the United Kingdom; the sad fact is that nearly all of these deaths can be prevented if the correct treatment is started early enough. Often, as the shortness of breath seems initially to be a minor symptom, it is ignored and action is not taken until far too late. The main aim of this book is to set out a simple, effective plan for coping with your child's asthma which is easy to follow and can be quickly put into effect. This plan has been built up and modified over the years both in my medical practice and my own home. The confidence it will give you will quickly be passed on to your child, so that much of the fear will very soon be taken out of the situation.

The management of asthma can be broadly divided into two sections: how to prevent the attacks starting; and how to cure them once the wheezing is established. We all hope that our children will grow out of their asthma as they become older, but research has shown this will only happen if the wheezing episodes can be kept to a minimum. In other words the longer the time interval between attacks the less likelihood there is of another one developing. Some children seem to have a slight wheeze nearly all the time and unless steps are taken to relieve this, there is no chance of a spontaneous remission. I remember Ross, one of my own sons, being short of breath continuously for nearly a month and how worried my wife and I became. Eventually his chest cleared but we were determined that he would never suffer like that again. Our knowledge and experience gained at that time formed the basis of the section of this book devoted to prevention.

Most of the methods of prevention can be applied to all children with asthma, but obviously there will be some individual variation, depending partly on the severity of the condition and also on differences in age and personality. Whereas one child could be settled with a straightforward change of diet, another might require the addition of an inhaler as well. The section on prevention has been built up step by step, starting with the simple guidelines and building up to more complex ones. Following these will mean you will not end up with your child on more treatment than is absolutely necessary. The treatment of an actual wheezing attack is also developed in stages, from a mild attack through to when the child is in a desperate condition. One of the major dangers in asthma is that only slight shortness of breath can deteriorate very rapidly into severe breathing difficulties. How to recognize when this may happen, and the methods of dealing with it, are clearly outlined.

In addition to the main chapters on treatment I have also included one on special situations, including exercise and holidays. In the surgery there are many questions that parents would like to ask but are prevented from doing so because the consultation time is too short. The chapter gives the answers to all the queries that have been raised by my own patients in the past year and includes additional ones that I have thought of myself when dealing with my asthmatic children at home.

Many people do not like the thought of long-term medication, and more and more are turning to natural therapies. As a GP with a keen interest in complementary medicine I have recommended natural methods wherever possible. However, as these tend to be slower in onset and more gradual in action, the rapidity of the asthma may be too fast for them to work on some occasions, and conventional medicine is then preferable. My own experience is that natural therapy is more effective when used in the prevention of attacks and for treatment of mild wheezing episodes.

The views and feelings of children themselves are often completely ignored when managing asthma, and often they can tell instinctively if the treatment is working and which type suits them best. I have included the children's own thoughts during wheezing episodes, as well as their opinions on the different types of therapy. Taking notice of children's comments has enabled me to make adjustments to my approach that I would not otherwise have realized were necessary. A simple example is the use of the inhaler called Ventolin. This is often stopped both by doctors and parents as it can cause a tremor of the hands; but this shaking rarely causes children any distress, and so often they lose a most effective medication on account of a harmless side-effect.

Throughout this book I have followed the progress of two young patients of mine, Simon and Julie, describing how they have dealt with the various stages of asthma and the difficulties they have experienced. I hope you will be able to see features of your own child in one of them. Where needed I have also included other children, as well as my own experiences with my asthmatic trio at home.

The book is designed to be one of action rather than theory, and it describes a plan for relieving asthma which I know is effective, and will bring much needed relief to both children and parents. I realize, however, that when your child becomes wheezy and short of breath the last thing you will do is to sit down and calmly read a book on the subject. Panic does tend to set in, and for this reason I have drawn easy-to-follow flow charts which will indicate the necessary treatment for the particular situation. A reference chart is given on page 156. When time is short and your brain is refusing to function coherently, it will be easier to assess the correct course of action.

CHAPTER 2

What is Asthma?

Julie is a young patient of mine who experienced her first serious asthma attack one evening when she was 4 years old. I remember visiting the following morning when her breathing had settled and Julie's parents were able to relax. Neither of them had ever seen anything as frightening before and naturally they asked me to explain the condition to them. It is important to understand what asthma means, its causes and the sequence of events that take place. This knowledge makes it much easier to establish an effective plan for prevention and treatment for your child.

Asthma is a condition affecting the airways of the lungs; the main function of the lungs is to breathe air in and out of the body. Every time Julie inhales, a certain amount of air passes through her mouth and nose into a single tube called the windpipe. This descends downwards into the chest where it divides into the right and left lungs. The bronchial tubes, as they are termed medically, then gradually divide a further twenty five times until they reach all parts of the lungs. At its top end the windpipe is about 2 cm wide and at the extremities the width is reduced to about half a millimetre. This layout is clearly shown in Figure 2.1.

The bronchial tubes are not rigid like metal pipes, but soft and kept open by muscles in the walls. Unfortunately these muscles are not like the muscles in our legs, as we cannot move them of our own free will; if irritated they tend to involuntarily contract. This squeezes the breathing tubes resulting in a narrowing of the hollow area inside, and a consequent reduction in the amount of air which can move through them. The medical term for this narrowing is broncho-constriction.

I explained to Julie's parents that their daughter's airways were more twitchy than normal. The reason for this is unknown and may well be some form of development problem before birth. If Julie is then exposed to certain trigger factors the muscles in the bronchi will contract violently, causing marked narrowing of the airways. These trigger factors vary from child to child, although dust and pollen are the commonest. The situation is further complicated by the fact that the bronchi have a delicate inner lining which can become swollen if irritated. In addition this lining secretes a fluid called mucus or phlegm which can clog up the breathing tubes.

In summary, the breathing tubes in an asthmatic child such as Julie become narrowed both by contraction of the outer muscle tissue and by swelling of the inner lining, with an excess amount of phlegm further worsening the situation. This is shown in Figure 2.2.

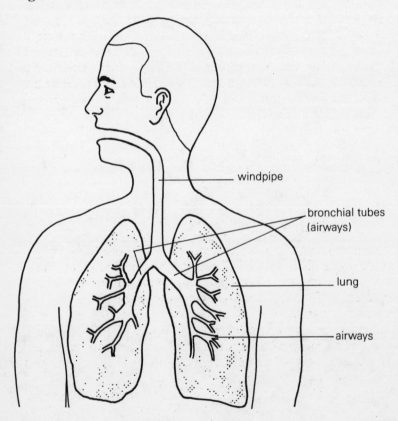

Figure 2.1   Diagram of airways

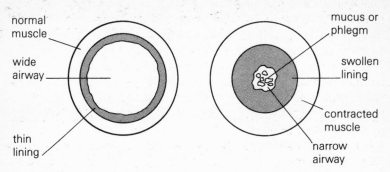

Figure 2.2   The effect of asthma on the bronchial tubes

Obviously, once the narrowing of the bronchi reaches a certain severity it becomes difficult to breath in enough oxygen or blow out sufficient carbon dioxide, and this makes the child short of breath. As I stressed to Julie's parents, at the start of an asthma attack it is only the muscle contraction that is important, as the swelling of the lining takes a few hours to develop. Therefore the earlier the asthma is diagnosed the less complex it is to treat and the quicker it will settle.

How to Recognize an Asthma Attack

While the theory of asthma is easy to understand, it is equally important to be able to recognize an attack in practice, so treatment can be commenced rapidly. No doubt some people reading this book will be well aware of how it affects their child, but others may not be so certain. Asthma can present in two different ways: as a chronic low-grade shortness of breath; or as a severe breathlessness of much faster onset. These are well illustrated by another two patients of mine, Richard and Simon.

Richard's mother had become increasingly worried about her 12 year-old son as he kept arriving home from school in a miserable state. He had always enjoyed playing football but recently had lost all enthusiasm for it. To make matters worse at a parents meeting she was told that Richard was falling behind with his schoolwork. He denied that anything was wrong and on several occasions had been angry with his mother for keeping on

> 1. Persistent cough — worse on exertion and at night
> 2. Wheezing and shortness of breath
> 3. General fall-off in performance

Table 2.1: Three main symptoms of asthma

at him about it. She decided that it was probably a phase he was going through, although lately he did seem to be coughing more than usual at night. Richard had tended to be 'chesty' when he was younger, and had often been given antibiotics by his GP. Matters came to a head one day when Richard was asked to rush to the post office to send off an urgent letter. He arrived home, very short of breath saying that he had just missed the post, at which his father became very annoyed because of the importance of the letter. Richard was very upset and over the next hour he became increasingly short of breath and distressed. His parents were worried when his breathing became noisy and he started to wheeze, so they called me out to visit.

Richard's main symptoms were a persistent cough, wheezing and a fall-off of performance, all of which are very typical of chronic asthma. (See Table 2.1 above.) Happily after examining him I was able to instigate the appropriate treatment using an inhaler and his breathing difficulty quickly settled.

I have found with my own three children that a troublesome cough is a warning that an asthma attack is threatened, and a sign temporarily to increase their medication. However, I am often asked by parents whether there is a single symptom which will confirm that their child has asthma - that sign is undoubtedly 'wheezing'.

In asthma there is more difficulty breathing out than breathing in. This is mainly because during inhalation there is a pull on the airways which tends to widen them. During expiration the reverse is true and the airways become relatively narrower. The child, therefore, in an attempt to breathe out sufficiently has to try and expel the air through the narrowed tubes. This produces the characteristic whistling sound known as a wheeze. In listening to Richard's breathing it was easy to see that inhaling was quite comfortable but each exhalation was prolonged, required much more effort, and was accompanied by the typical wheeze. This one feature is itself virtually diagnostic of asthma.

Richard's attacks were low-grade ones which built up over a period of several weeks. Simon, however – in similar fashion to Julie – developed a much more sudden and savage attack during a freezing winter night. He had suffered from a common cold for the previous three days but this was not unusual as his mother commented that he always picked infections up very easily. He was now 10 years old and this was the first time he had been in such distress. When I arrived, to a very worried household, Simon was sat up in a chair and looked extremely ill. The dominant feature was the violent wheezing with severe shortness of breath. He was pale and his facial expression was anxious with beads of sweat on his brow. He was cold to the touch, with a clammy skin. His heartbeat was very fast and increased every time he tried to force a breath in. The soft tissues around his neck and the muscles between his ribs were sucked in every time he inhaled. Simon was sitting forward with his elbows on his knees gasping for breath. Speech was almost non-existent save for short phrases, and he was extremely restless.

At this stage it is almost impossible to reassure either child or parents and management is aimed solely at relieving the breathing difficulty. Up to a few years ago this would have meant admission to hospital, but apart from causing further anxiety, vital minutes would be lost before treatment was started; the wait for an ambulance, even though they come quickly, can seem to last for an eternity and many is the time I have taken an asthmatic child up to hospital in my own car.

Fortunately a great deal of progress has been made in the treatment of these severe attacks, and now, with the use of a machine called a nebulizer, relief can be obtained very rapidly. Simon used the nebulizer for ten minutes and it became possible for him to breathe out more freely. He still had a wheeze but it was not so forced. In only a short space of time the tension relaxed and the mood of the whole house was lifted. It took Simon another twenty-four hours to become free of his wheeze, but during this time he was quite happy and was able to move about virtually as normal.

In all three of the cases I have just described the parents were most anxious to know the cause of the attacks and whether they could be prevented. I will discuss this in the next chapter.

CHAPTER 3

The Causes of Asthma

A cardinal rule in any illness is to identify its underlying cause, because only then can specific treatment be given. In asthma the wheezing is produced by narrowing of the bronchial airways, mainly caused by muscle spasm in the walls of the tubes. The degree of this constriction determines whether the child has only minor symptoms or has extreme shortness of breath. But what causes this muscle to narrow in the first place?

It has been well proven that there are certain stimuli that will provide tightening of the airways. These are:

- ALLERGY
- EMOTION
- POLLUTION
- INFECTION
- EXERTION

Why, however, do these trigger factors not cause asthma in every child? The reason is that some children have an underlying general irritability of their breathing tubes, which means that the tubes constrict very easily on exposure to one of, or a combination of, these factors. This is undoubtedly an inherited trait which is present before birth and shows itself predominantly in the first ten years of life. After that age, the airways gradually become less sensitive and the child then 'grows out' of the asthma. Sometimes the bronchial muscles are so irritable that not only do they react to the inhaling of major stimuli but also to the accidental breathing of simple irritants like cold air and smoke. Even such commonplace disturbances as laughter or exercise can be followed in the asthmatic child by an embarrassing wheezing and tightness in the chest.

If you can identify which of these factors produce wheezing attacks in your own child then it is quite possible either to avoid them or dampen them down in some way so as to prevent the asthma starting. A few children are only sensitive to one of these groups, but more commonly it is a combination. Exposure to only a single stimulant may not be sufficient to create problems but as soon as another is thrown in, then the attack will start.

Before looking at these causes in more detail let us first consider 10 year-old Simon, one of the children described in the previous chapter. Simon's first major attack was a severe one in the middle of the night, but talking to his parents produced some interesting information about Simon's prior symptoms. For the past three summers Simon had suffered quite marked hay fever, which is a condition produced by an allergy to pollen. His mother commented that he tended to worry about things, especially returning to school after the holidays. If he ever caught a cold he would have a troublesome cough for some weeks which was much worse if he was in a smoky atmosphere. During games periods Simon sometimes had to stop to catch his breath.

If we look for the precipitating causes for his actual asthma attack, it is easy to see that Simon has a sensitivity to all the main groups of trigger factors; he has an allergy to pollen, is very emotional, has a persistent cough when in a polluted atmosphere or following a cold, and becomes short of breath on exertion. I suppose it is surprising therefore that Simon did not have a serious bout of asthma before the age of 10.

Four year-old Julie, who I also described in Chapter 2, had suffered with eczema since she was a baby and seemed to have a constant runny nose. Eczema at this age is nearly always allergic in nature, and the repeated infections in her nose did not - as in most children - clear up in a couple of days, but always left her with an irritating cough. Thus Julie had only two of the major causes of asthma, i.e. allergy and infection, but they were still sufficient to give her a severe bout of wheezing.

Allergy

Both sets of parents were very keen to look into the precise causes of their children's asthma in more detail, in particular the allergy factor. Simon's father pointed out to me that although Simon suffered badly from hay fever, which is a pollen allergy,

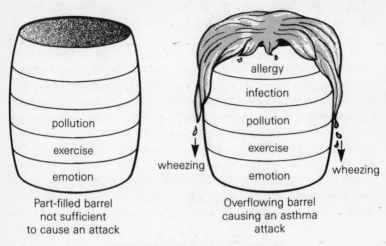

Figure 3.1   'The asthma barrel'

this only occurred in summer, whereas his asthma attack was in winter. I explained that anyone with an allergy to one substance is nearly always allergic to many different ones. Some of these on their own do not produce any symptoms, but when thinking about asthma it is useful to imagine an empty barrel into which the child's different allergies are being thrown. No trouble occurs until the barrel is full, and it may take many allergens together to reach this point. If another allergic substance is then tossed into the barrel it overflows and problems immediately begin, which in the case of asthma is wheezing and shortness of breath. (See Figure 3.1.)

An allergic reaction is an abnormal response to a substance which has no effect on normal or non-allergic people. The problem is identifying the factors to which your own child is allergic. While there are hundreds of substances that can cause a reaction, it is often quite easy to identify the ones producing the strongest effect.

Nearly all asthmatic children are allergic to the house-dust mite. This is a tiny insect which lives in household dust, and is invisible to the naked eye. Mites are most dangerous on the mattress when the child is in bed inhaling the allergen all night. Although the mite is also present in the carpet, children do not tend to lie with their faces buried in the carpet for any length of time.

Pollen is another substance which can produce a strong

allergic reaction leading to asthma. In the height of summer there is a tremendous amount of pollen released into the air. If a child who is allergic to pollen walks through a field where grass is freshly cut then he or she will inhale a large quantity of pollen grains. As these enter the lungs they provoke coughing, wheezing and shortness of breath. An identical situation can arise from the inhalation of animal danders, a mixture of fur, hair, scale and urine shed from pets. Dogs, cats and horses are the animals most commonly implicated.

It is easy to understand how something which is inhaled directly into the lungs can produce a reaction in the breathing tubes. Asthma can also develop from allergic substances which are eaten or drunk. The foods most commonly incriminated are cow's milk, eggs, wheat, cheese, yeast, fish, pork and peanuts. Unfortunately the picture is further complicated by the preservatives and colourants used by food manufacturers. Many asthmatic children are allergic to the tartrazine in orange squash and cola and in some the reaction is strong enough to make them wheeze.

Sometimes a little detective work is needed to identify your child's allergies, but this will be very rewarding if it lessens the frequency and severity of the attacks.

The Major Allergic Factors

Inhaled	Consumed
House-dust mite	Cow's milk
Animal fur	Orange squash (Tartrazine)
Pollen	Nuts
Moulds and spores	Dairy produce
Feathers	Fish
	Pork

In my experience nearly every asthmatic child is allergic in varying degrees to all the inhaled allergens and to certain of the consumed ones. Simon had always been upset by cheese and orange squash, and Julie was particularly affected by milk and cola. We shall consider dealing with these allergic factors in the section on prevention.

Emotion

Let me say at the outset that I am a firm believer in the theory that emotional upsets in a child can trigger an asthma attack.

Until very recently it has been widely accepted within medical circles that asthmatics were rather emotional types who could easily develop an attack when distressed. This was always said in a rather critical way as if inferring the child was a 'weakling'. This opinion I am certain originates from people who have never had first-hand experience of looking after an asthmatic child. My own son, Ross (as in the case of Simon described above) is a very tough boy, but he tends to be a worrier. All through the school holidays he will be perfectly calm with little or no problem with his breathing. Two days before school all that changes as he starts to worry about going back. Within a few hours he starts to wheeze and become short of breath. In other words, it isn't the asthma that produces the upset – it is the exact reverse. This does not make Ross a 'weakling' in any way but it does make him the type in whom stress can produce an asthma attack.

Pollution

This category is extremely important in triggering wheezing episodes. On many occasions I have been called out to see children with asthma only to have to fight my way through a cloud of cigarette smoke to reach them. An irritant atmosphere is deadly to a child's lungs, and it amazes me that so many parents will subject their children to such torture. In fact I now carry round with me a small machine which analyses the amount of smoke in the air so I can show parents the high levels only one cigarette can produce.

Other pollutants that are harmful to the lungs include the smoke from coal fires, industrial smog, and car exhaust fumes.

Infection

'When he catches a cold it goes straight on his chest.' This is a frequent comment from parents and undoubtedly it occurs with certain types of infection. It is most important to distinguish viral infections from bacterial ones, as it is the former that produce the wheezing. The common cold is produced by a virus and this then irritates the airways, producing an asthma attack. Other infections, like tonsillitis, sinusitis, and pneumonia, are caused by different bugs called bacteria – but these for some reason do not irritate the chest. It is important to understand this as antibiotics will kill bacteria but not viruses. Antibiotics therefore have absolutely no part to play in the treatment of asthma and should not be looked upon as necessary or beneficial either by doctors or parents.

Exertion

This may seem a strange cause, as even the fittest among us will become short of breath during exercise. The difference is that in non-asthmatics when the exertion is stopped the airways quickly settle back to normal. In asthma sufferers this is not so. The breathing tubes reach their narrowest between three and five minutes later, remaining at that level for some time after. In other words the shortness of breath actually increases when exercise is stopped. Different sports are more harmful than others and running is certainly the worst. Wheezing when exercising may occur in asthmatic children within six to eight minutes, and this can be very hazardous in a cross-country run at school. Cycling induces asthma although not so consistently, perhaps because only the legs are used. Other factors, like a cold wind and exhaust fumes, may play a contributory part in asthma caused by cycling. Swimming seems to be the most innocuous of all and can be recommended to everyone. As a general rule light exercise is less likely to induce wheezing although a harder sport like football can be well tolerated provided it is in brief bursts with some respite in-between.

Almost all asthmatic children have wheezing with exercise but why this should occur is a mystery. It is thought that it must be due to the release of some chemical in the lungs that affects the muscles in the airways. This is really of little practical help at this stage, but hopefully in the future it may be possible to identify and reverse the effect of this substance.

Simon's first attempt at cross-country running was a disaster, as he had to give up on the second lap. This was most upsetting to him as he didn't want to appear 'soft' to the rest of his classmates, and his teacher thought he was not really trying. It was only when he saw Simon in considerable distress a few minutes after stopping that he realized how serious the condition had become. Simon's parents wanted him to be able to do everything that normal children can do and naturally this is the aim of treatment in all asthmatic children.

By accurately identifying the causes of your child's asthma it is quite easy to take the necessary steps to deal with them. This chapter has shown the major trigger factors and it is nearly always one or a combination of these that produce the attacks. If you have not been able to identify the specific problems in your own child do not despair; by moving on to the plan for prevention and treatment I am certain that complete control of this troublesome condition can be obtained.

CHAPTER 4

Tests for Asthma in Children

The diagnosis of asthma is usually made from the appearance of a wheezy, distressed child who is short of breath. Both the children featured in the previous chapters, Simon and Julie, presented in this manner and as soon as I saw them the diagnosis was obvious. Even if the symptoms are less severe the child's description of them is usually accurate enough to confirm the diagnosis. However, on some occasions, doubts may still linger in both doctor's and parents' minds, and certain tests may then be arranged by your GP. The test can have three functions: to confirm the diagnosis of asthma; to rule out other possible types of chest problems; and in some cases to try and determine the underlying cause of the attacks.

Blood Tests

These are carried out on a small sample of blood from the child's arm, and only need to be performed at the initial examination. The tests check there are sufficient cells present in the blood to fight infections. One particular constituent is the white blood cell, which destroys invading viruses and bacteria and forms part of the body's natural defence system, known as the immune system. There are many millions of these present in every pint of blood. In asthmatic children there may be a marked reduction in these particular cells, leaving the children more prone to infections.

Our blood also contains certain proteins; the levels of one such protein, called IgE, are raised if the person is highly allergic. Children with asthma are therefore more likely to have high IgE levels, and these will show on the laboratory test.

Chest X-Ray

Parents often think that chest X-rays are vital in the diagnosis of asthma, but it is important to realize that in nearly all children the X-ray will be completely normal. The main reason for taking a film is to exclude other, less common causes of wheezing. One possibility is cystic fibrosis which is a rare condition in which the lungs become clogged with thick mucus. Alternatively a small object like a peanut may have been inhaled straight into the lungs. This classically happens when the nut is thrown into the air and caught in the mouth, for at this angle the peanut may pass straight down the windpipe. Chest X-rays may also be of help where an infection is present at the same time as the asthma, as the extent and severity of the affected area shows up clearly.

Lung Function Tests

Children can be tested for asthma by breathing into a machine which monitors how effectively the lungs are working. The simplest of these is a small calibrated plastic tube, called a peak flow meter. This measures the amount of air that a child can blow out of the lungs in one second. As the airways are narrowed in asthma, it follows that less air can be blown out through them. Thus if they are half their normal width then only half the amount of air can be expelled at each breath. This measurement is recorded by the peak flow meter, which plays a major role in the management of asthma and is discussed in much greater detail in the section on prevention (see pp.37–8). It is a useful tool in diagnosing asthma as the initial reading may be much lower than would be expected even in the absence of significant wheezing.

Allergy Tests

All asthmatic children suffer from allergies, although some are more severe than others. It would seem logical to try to identify these allergens, sc they can be avoided. The commonest method available is skin testing, which involves placing a drop of liquid on the arm and pricking the skin through the drop with a small needle. In the liquid is an extract of a particularly allergic substance, for example house dust. If the child has an allergy to this then an itchy red weal will form around the pin-prick, and the size of this weal is a reflection of how strong the allergy is to that particular trigger factor. Usually about six tests are carried out at the same time and normally include house-dust mite, feathers, dog and cat danders, grass and tree pollens. These can be added to if there is anything the parents think the child may be allergic to; nowadays skin tests can be prepared for virtually any chemical.

The usefulness of allergy tests is well illustrated by 10 year-old Suzie, who had never previously had any breathing problems. She was very keen to start horse-riding, but after a couple of lessons noticed a tickly cough and a tight sensation in her chest. The next week Suzie became a little short of breath when running to catch the horse. Then after a vigorous grooming and brushing session she became obviously wheezy and distressed. At the surgery I carried out a skin test with horse hair extract which produced a large red weal indicating a strongly positive allergy to horses. As it happened Suzie's keen desire to learn riding had lessened so she decided to give it up rather than go through a course of desensitizing injections.

The allergies discussed above are all caused by inhaled substances which act directly on the lungs. However, there is a group of allergens which occur in food and drink which is thought to be responsible for between 10 and 20 per cent of all childhood asthma. The foods most commonly incriminated are dairy products including cow's milk and cheese, eggs, wheat, yeast, fish, pork and nuts. Some children are sensitive to colourants and preservatives used by food manufacturers, and without doubt there has been an increase in the number of asthma cases caused by these in the past few years.

Mark was a 9 year-old boy who had always had a finicky appetite, periods of irritability, poor sleep and difficulty in concentration at school. This combined with his asthma suggested a food allergy. On asking about his diet Mark's father remarked that he liked to drink plenty of orange squash and cola. The tartrazine in both these drinks is a well known allergen and on omitting both squash and cola all Mark's symptoms greatly improved. On one occasion he did have a glass of squash at a party and this was followed quite quickly by a wheezing episode.

The difficulty with food allergies is identifying them accurately. Skin tests are occasionally useful but more often than not only a trial diet to avoid various foods will confirm a sensitivity. This can be a problem because it may be several weeks before the allergy dies down. An example of this is dairy produce which can take up to six weeks before the airways settle. How to manage food allergies is discussed at greater length in the section on prevention (see pp. 44–6, 54).

Now that I have described the tests available let us see how they were applied to our two main cases in this book, Simon and Julie. Let us consider Julie first. We discovered in Chapter 3 that Julie had two main groups of trigger factors; she had long-standing eczema of the skin which strongly suggested allergies, and any cold or sore throats were often followed by wheezing, indicating that infection was a major precipitant of her asthma. Her parents were both very keen to try and pinpoint the causes for her asthma and actually asked if Julie could have a chest X-ray.

Initially I took a small sample of blood from her arm, which Julie was not too happy about but I assured her it would help us in identifying the reason for her wheezing. Fortunately the levels of the different blood cells were normal, although her IgE level was raised, which confirmed she suffered from allergies. Her mother was worried that the colds were causing infection to spread on to Julie's chest, so a chest X-ray was arranged at the local hospital. The specialist's report indicated the lungs were completely normal in appearance with no evidence of any infection or other condition. I carried out simple lung function tests in the surgery using a peak flow meter and this confirmed some reduction in the passages of air in and out of the lungs. Julie had a cat and dog as pets so these were included in her skin tests. The six tests carried out were to grass pollen, feathers, house-dust mite, and dog, cat and horse hair. All six showed a positive reaction, particularly pollen, feathers and house-dust mite. Julie was very pleased that her pets were not the main problem as they would definitely have been under threat of expulsion!

Before considering the meaning of these test results let us first consider Simon's situation. We had established in Chapter 3 that the main trigger factors were allergies, emotion, exertion, cold winds and pollution in the atmosphere. His parents felt that their son had gone through a great deal with his asthma and were not at all keen for him to have any tests performed unless they were completely necessary. The diagnosis of asthma was not in doubt as I had seen Simon in a severe attack. On clinical examination he was a good healthy colour so it was most unlikely that a blood test would show up any deficiency. We were already aware that he suffered from hay fever so his blood would be sure to be positive anyway for allergies.

Between attacks his chest was completely clear and there had never been any sign of infection on his chest. Although I suggested a chest X-ray his mum said she wasn't keen on him having any unnecessary radiation. As far as identifying the allergens by skin-testing I must admit they are not particularly pleasant for the child and Simon always in the past had become most upset at the sight of a needle. We already knew from his hay fever that he would show positive to grass and tree pollen. His mother had previously changed from feather pillows to synthetic and he didn't have any pets. Furthermore I had to admit that I haven't yet seen an asthmatic child who hasn't shown positive allergic reactions to house-dust mite. So, in fact the only test that Simon had was one for lung function and he quite enjoyed blowing into this small machine. It was easy to demonstrate that he had marked reduction in airflow, which was accentuated after a simple exercise of jogging on the spot for a few minutes.

Simon and Julie represent the two extremes when it comes to testing for asthma with Julie having virtually all of them and Simon only one! In the early part of this chapter I described all the tests that are available for asthma and many doctors and specialists do still carry out all of them as a sort of blanket investigation. However, some of the procedures, particularly anything to do with needles, are not going to be popular with the child.

So which ones are really necessary? Much depends on how much confidence and faith you have in your own doctor. Actually diagnosing asthma in a child is not difficult for anyone with medical training and does not really need any tests to confirm it. While Julie's parents accepted their daughter suffered from asthma they had experienced problems with their previous GP so were not keen to rely purely on my opinion. They were quite happy therefore for Julie to have all the tests. In Simon's case I had looked after the family for many years and had been present at his birth. The family therefore were quite happy with my conclusions so did not want tests carried out merely to confirm what I had already pointed out.

To Test or Not to Test

If you are not sure which to have, let us briefly go through the different tests again and I will explain my personal feelings on them. If your child is fit and active between attacks I can't see a particular reason for a routine blood test. It is unpleasant to have done and there is no real gain. While it will demonstrate the presence of allergy it won't identify which particular allergen is the criminal. As all asthmatic children have allergies it doesn't really contribute very much to the management.

Chest infections play no part in the production of an asthma attack so in my mind there is no place for a chest X-ray. The only exception is if your doctor wants to exclude uncommon conditions like cystic fibrosis. Please do not worry about this because it is extremely rare. Not only that but your child would be quite ill and it is not usually necessary to confirm it by X-ray.

Skin tests *en bloc* do not necessarily provide useful information as often the asthmatic child is positive to every allergen tested. As I pointed out above I have never seen a child with asthma who wasn't allergic to house-dust mite and pollen. Where they are particularly useful is in testing for a specific allergy, like Suzie's allergy to horses. Often the household pets are thought to be the problem but it is important to have positive proof before considering any drastic action.

Lung function tests are vital because not only do they confirm the diagnosis but they show the degree of the condition in everyday life.

So, the most important point in asthma testing is to be selective for your own child. The only essential investigation is that of lung function though selective skin testing can be most valuable. This to me seems a more sensible approach than subjecting your child to unnecessary trauma.

Prevention of Asthma Attacks

'Can't you stop me having these attacks, Daddy?' pleaded my little daughter Tina on one occasion when she was particularly breathless and was unable to go to school. It would have to be the one time when her class was going on an outing which Tina had been looking forward to for several weeks. Not only that but my wife had commented about ten days previously that the wheezing episodes seemed to be coming much more frequently and this was the fourth day in a month that Tina would miss a day at school. Certainly her actual attacks were being effectively treated but the methods we were using to prevent them were obviously totally inadequate.

It is most distressing to see your own child fighting for breath so it is vital to use all possible means to avert this happening, provided this does not interfere with the quality of life. All asthmatics should be able to lead a normal life and take part in all the usual activities without fear of becoming wheezy. In this section therefore we will look at the different methods of prevention, how effective they are and how they form part of a practical plan.

Prevention can be divided into four basic principles:

1. Ensure the natural body defences or immune system are in tip-top condition.
2. Where possible, remove any obvious causes of the asthma attacks.
3. Regularly use any medication that has been prescribed.
4. Investigate the alternative methods of control, e.g. relaxation techniques, breathing exercises, homoeopathy, acupuncture and hypnosis.

CHAPTER 5

Prevention Using Inhaled Medication

Asthma is a serious and potentially life-threatening condition. Over the years medical research has developed drugs which are both safe and effective in preventing the attacks occurring. It may seem strange therefore that the number of hospital admissions – and indeed deaths – is still increasing each year. I am certain the main reason is that parents are reluctant to let their children take medication on a regular basis because of the fear of side-effects. While this is generally an excellent principle, in asthma the situation is different. If a wheezing episode is prevented then not only does it save the child tremendous suffering but it also means that the much stronger drugs which must be used in an attack will not be necessary.

Let us consider the two children we have followed so far through this book, Julie, aged 4, and Simon who is 10. Following her severe attack Julie's parents were very concerned that it might happen again – they had been convinced at one stage that their daughter's life was in danger. However, they were worried about any harmful effects of continuous therapy and asked me to explain the situation fully to them. Fortunately modern drug development has enabled the present preventive medicine to be breathed directly into the lungs using a small device called an inhaler – commonly known as a 'puffer'. Until this technique was perfected, all anti-asthma drugs had to be given either in medicine or tablet form. These would be ingested in the stomach before passing into the bloodstream and would then travel through every part of the body, producing their various unwanted effects before finally arriving at the lungs. For this reason these drugs were slow to work and often associated with unpleasant side-effects. Contrast this with the newer medications which are inhaled directly to the trouble spot so

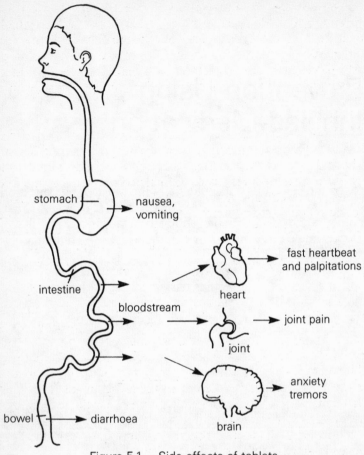

Figure 5.1   Side-effects of tablets

their mode of action is very fast. As they are not absorbed into the rest of the body there are almost no adverse effects. (See Figure 5.1.)

I reminded Julie's parents that there were two main changes in the lungs during an asthma attack. Firstly there is a tightening - or spasm - of the muscles in the breathing tubes, and secondly the lining of these tubes becomes swollen. The effect of both of these factors is to make the airways much narrower, so the child becomes short of breath and wheezy. The preventive medication that has been developed is aimed at stopping this spasm and swelling from developing. It may not be necessary for your own child to have both forms of treatment; in Julie's case

I suggested she should start on an inhaler only to stop the spasm. Particularly effective is a substance known as Intal which must be taken between two and four times a day. When this was discovered it completely revolutionized the management of asthma as here was a method of controlling the condition without the risk of side-effects. It is taken through a special kind of inhaler called a 'spinhaler'.

Intal is a dry powder, and a measured dose is contained in a small plastic capsule. This is inserted into the spinhaler (see Figure 5.2) and is punctured by sliding a small cutting device. The end of the inhaler is then placed in the child's mouth and when the next breath is taken the Intal powder is sucked into the lungs. I showed Julie how to do this but as often happens in young children she was not very keen at first. This reluctance was easily overcome by attaching a whistle to the end of the spinhaler so when she inhaled a loud whistling sound was produced. Naturally this was great fun and all her previous inhibitions were soon forgotten!

By using this Intal spinhaler three times a day Julie was able easily to control her asthma. Her mother asked how long it would be necessary for Julie to stay on this treatment and I warned both her parents never to become complacent about this condition. The problem with being well controlled is that it is difficult to tell whether the child has grown out of the asthma or if the improvement is solely a result of treatment. It is vital therefore never to stop Intal suddenly, and I usually recommend six months to a year of continuous use, free from attacks, before a reduction is made. Even then it is important to reduce the doses in stages.

Generally Intal is very easy to use, but one of the difficulties I found at home with my children was that if the capsules

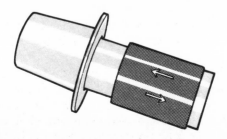

Figure 5.2   A spinhaler

became damp, the cutting device in the spinhaler would not puncture the plastic. The design does not allow you to see if this has happened and sometimes my son Ross would become exasperated when sucking away at his inhaler only to find nothing coming out! There is no option when this happens but to go back to your doctor for another prescription. The capsules are supplied in a damp-proof container, but children tend to forget and leave the top loose which allows the moisture to seep in.

Simon's attacks were much more frequent than Julie's and although he responded well to Intal his father thought he still had a tendency to wheeze at times, especially at night. It seemed that Simon, as well as having marked spasm of his breathing tubes, also had a degree of swelling of their linings. For this I recommended adding the other type of preventive inhaler which contains a steroid. His parents immediately expressed dismay at the thought of this as they had heard of some of the less desirable effects steroids can have on the body. While it is true that when taken by mouth for long periods of time they can affect growth in children, this is not so in the inhaled form. As I have mentioned the real benefit of inhaling a medication straight into the lungs is that it is not absorbed into the rest of the body so side-effects do not occur. Steroids given in this way are therefore harmless.

This inhaler, the commonest of which is called Becotide 50, is different to the spinhaler in that it is a pressurized aerosol, and it is not necessary to insert a capsule as the powder is already contained in the barrel of the inhaler itself. By inserting one end into the mouth and as you breathe in pressing the bottom a set dose of medication is released and automatically inhaled. This is much easier than 'messing about' putting in a capsule but there are two potential disadvantages. First, it is necessary to ensure that the inhaler is activated just as you are breathing in or else the powder will not pass to the lungs. This is extremely important, and as inhalers are used throughout the treatment of asthma I have included a special chapter on inhaler technique (see p. 80). Second, even using the correct method the powder may come out with such force that some of it will hit the back of the throat and not go into the lungs. However, even with these drawbacks it is still a most effective treatment and in Simon's case the simple addition of two puffs twice a day stopped the underlying wheeze.

So now we can start to build up our complete treatment plan which is shown in Figure 5.3 below. We know that to prevent an asthma attack we should first use Intal and add Becotide if it is ineffective. Sometimes if there is still insufficient control it may be necessary to increase the strength of the steroid to Becotide 100. Very occasionally children are unable to use the inhaler correctly and then it may be necessary to change to a diskhaler where the steroid is in powder form. This is sucked into the lungs as they breathe in but does not rely on co-ordinating breathing in with operating the device. The disadvantage is the same as for Intal, i.e. special discs containing the powder have to be loaded into the diskhaler.

Although delighted at their respective children's improvements, both sets of parents were worried as to how they could tell in the very early stages if the preventive treatment is insufficient. Obviously it is easy to tell if the child starts to wheeze but it would be much better if an impending asthma attack could be diagnosed some time before the wheeze starts. In general the quicker the treatment is started the faster the attack will settle. The easiest way of telling is by the appearance of an irritating cough, which means the airways are becoming twitchy and may soon tighten up. In my own three children, especially Ross and Tina, the cough is very pronounced and gives us about two hours to reverse the situation before the shortness of breath begins.

However, this cough is not always present and a far more active way of showing that problems with breathing are starting is by the use of a peak flow meter. This is a small portable plastic device which in essence measures the amount of air which can

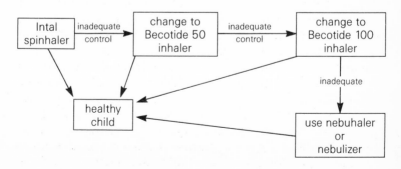

Figure 5.3   Complete treatment plan – prevention

A mini-Wright peak flow meter

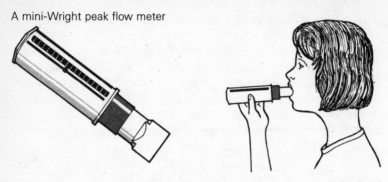

Figure 5.4   Peak flow meter

be forcibly blown out of the lungs (see Figure 5.4).

The peak flow meter is a vital piece of equipment and no child with asthma should be without one. They can now be obtained on prescription from your doctor. The end of the tube with the mouthpiece is placed between the lips and a deep breath in is taken. The child then breathes out as hard as possible and the force of this exhalation pushes a pointer up the scale. If the breathing tubes are tightening up, i.e. they are becoming narrower than normal, then the child will be unable to blow as much air into the peak flow meter and a lower reading on the scale will be produced. The measurement that can be achieved depends on age, height and sex, so it will vary for each child.

The readings are usually constant at a certain figure, and if they then start to decrease it indicates that the airways are starting to narrow and an asthma attack is on the way. In general the breathing tubes are naturally a little narrower at night than during the day, so another pointer is if this gap in readings between the morning and evening starts to widen. (This also explains why asthma attacks tend to be worse at night.)

At my own surgery I provide all asthmatic children with a record card to note down their peak flow readings every day, so it is possible to see their normal levels and detect whether any deterioration occurs. Although it may seem that wheezing attacks occur very suddenly, often there is a gradual deterioration in peak flow readings for several days before. If either the child or parents notice this reduction in levels then the appropriate action can be taken before the breathing becomes distressed.

Let us see how this is applied in practice to our two children Julie and Simon. The first important fact to establish was their normal healthy maximum peak flow meter score. Simon, who was the elder, reached a figure of 400 on the scale, and Julie who was smaller came to 250. The figure for your own child must be kept firmly in your head as a fall in peak flow readings often occurs for several hours before there is any feeling of wheezing or shortness of breath. In Simon's case I explained the general rules for dealing with a fall-off in levels:

- if the reduction does not go lower than 300, i.e. no more than 25 per cent below normal, then this can be easily managed at home and often only necessitates extra doses of preventive medication.
- if the reduction is down to the 200-300 range or around 50 per cent of normal then active treatment of an attack must be started as recommended in the main treatment chart.
- any score less than 200 means the asthma attack is becoming severe and it is wise to seek a doctor's help as well as instigating the treatment plan.
- if the reading falls below 100 then treatment is particularly urgent.

Simon was well controlled on Intal and Becotide inhalers, both on a twice daily dosage. However, on one occasion – when he was close to going back to school and therefore under stress – his parents noticed his peak flow readings were falling. They phoned me at the surgery when the readings reached 320 to ask what action they should take. Now it is important to be aggressive when treating asthma so I doubled the dose of both the spinhaler and the inhaler to four times daily. Gradually over the next couple of days his peak flow readings climbed back up to the normal level of 400. Here was an effective way to prevent an attack as a 25 per cent reduction in peak flow had not caused any problems with Simon's breathing. His parents were delighted as he would have developed a wheezing attack without the increase in treatment. They have used his peak flow meter on many occasions since, either to prevent an attack coming on or to judge the strength and type of treatment required.

Julie, being only 4, needed to use a smaller flow meter and it did take practice for her to become proficient at using it. However, it did prove very reliable and the same percentage reductions applied as with Simon. Her normal level was 250, so

Reading	Action needed
less than 25% reduction	increase Intal and Becotide inhalers
25–50% reduction	active treatment of attack
50–75% reduction	call doctor and initiate treatment for severe attack
more than 75% reduction	needs urgent hospital treatment — take direct to casualty department

Table 5.1: Reduction in peak flow

as long as the reading did not fall below 190 it only required an increase in her Intal. This happened on one occasion when she developed a cold and was the time she was most likely to develop an asthma attack. By increasing her Intal from three times a day to four her peak flow rapidaly improved.

So it can be clearly seen that if action is taken during the first reduction in peak flow readings, by increasing the preventive medication, then often an asthma attack can be averted. This is why a peak flow meter is absolutely essential in asthma as it picks up changes in airflow long before the child feels them.

Asthma in the Very Young

Wheezing attacks can occur in babies but this is usually harmless as attacks are only mild. However, asthma may develop from the age of 12 months onwards and at this age it can present a management problem, as babies cannot manage the inhaler. The main reason for this is they are unable to co-ordinate the breath in with pressing the bottom of the inhaler to release the spray. Not only that, but this spray comes out with such force that most of it hits the back of the throat and very little goes into the lungs.

Yvette was 14 months old and had suffered three wheezing episodes in two months and her parents were naturally very worried about any further attacks. As the inhalers cause such problems at this age it may be necessary to resort to medicine by mouth. The preparation with the least side-effects is Alupent which, if given in the dose of one teaspoon three times daily, will keep the airways open. The problem is that, as it affects the rest of the body as well as the lungs, the dose has to be kept at a low level. Yvette's mother was not keen on the idea of continuous medicine and asked if there was any other way of preventing the wheezing. The method of treatment I find most beneficial is to use a device called a volumatic or nebuhaler (see Figure 5.5). This is basically a large plastic container which fits on to an ordinary inhaler. Three puffs of the medication can then be squeezed into this container and the baby or young child can inhale it without having to worry about co-ordinating the breathing.

If the wheezing is still not fully controlled then the medication can be inhaled using a special machine called a nebulizer. This is an electrical device which turns the drug into a vapour which is then breathed in slowly over a period of ten minutes. The vapour is inhaled via a mask which can be held close to a baby's mouth. In older children it is usually only necessary to use this machine during an actual attack, and I have described this fully in the treatment section (see p. 107). Yvette settled very well with the use of a nebuhaler and managed with this until she was old enough to use the smaller inhaler. The only disadvantage of the nebuhaler is that it is bulky and cannot be carried around in a pocket or handbag. Figure 5.6 summarizes the prevention plan for babies.

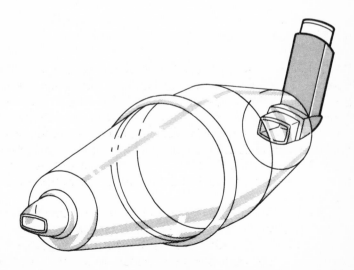

Figure 5.5   Nebuhaler

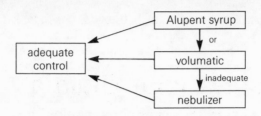

Figure 5.6   Summary of prevention plan for babies

Asthma Clinics

Different doctors will have their own particular ways of preventing and treating asthma attacks. In this book I am building up a method which I know works quickly and effectively with minimal upset to the child. Unfortunately, asthma can occur at any time of the day or night and it may be that the on-call doctor is used to dealing with wheezing in a different way. This can be most confusing to the parents. To avoid this happening many practices have started an asthma clinic, in which there is a common policy leading to consistent management. In other words, all children will be treated in the same way by each doctor. It also has the advantage that asthma sufferers can attend at any time if they feel all is not well. One of the major reasons for lack of control is poor inhaler technique and the clinics enable the practice nurse and doctor to correct this if necessary. Simon, who is the least stable of our cases, attended the clinic on several occasions when he was learning to use his inhalers.

If asthma is to be effectively prevented, then as well as no wheezing, there must be no night or morning coughing, no coughing with vigorous exercise, no coughing in cold air and no coughing with cigarette smoke. Only if these criteria are met can the preventive treatment be considered a success.

We can now continue to build up the complete management plan for asthma.

CHAPTER 6

Boosting your Child's Immune System

While the use of inhaled medication is the most popular way of preventing asthma, there are several other approaches which may be used as alternatives. Even if, on its own, each method may not be sufficient to completely prevent wheezing attacks, when used in combination they can reduce the amount and frequency of conventional drugs required. Despite all the advances in treatment through the years the most powerful protection against illness is still our own natural defence mechanism known as the immune system. When the body is challenged by anything foreign, whether it be an injury, a nasty little bug or an allergy, then this system immediately sets to work to heal the affected area. This is mainly achieved by special cells in the blood called lymphocytes, and many millions extra of these are produced at the first sign of ill health.

However, our immune systems also need looking after and if we do not keep them in excellent condition our body defences can become inefficient and ultimately may fail. I am sure there have been times when you have felt run down and it seems you catch all kinds of minor infections like repeated colds and sore throats. Cuts and grazes take longer to heal and often become septic. What is really happening is that your immune system is below par and is unable to fight off these minor conditions that normally it would deal with quite easily. In children the body defences are usually particularly strong but also are especially vulnerable if not kept in perfect condition.

So how does this apply to asthma? When your child catches a cold or is challenged by an allergy, these will not cause a major effect on the body, if the immune system is working efficiently. If the defences are 'down' these colds and allergens can take such a hold that an asthma attack develops.

It is vital therefore in any child who suffers from asthma to ensure that the immune system is in perfect condition at all times. But how can this be achieved? Basically there are three factors that suppress the natural defences: a poor diet; lack of exercise; and too little sleep and relaxation.

Diet in Children

'Wouldn't it be nice if I could always eat exactly what I want?' exclaimed my son Ross one lunchtime when he was none too happy about the meal before him. It certainly seems at times that everything we like is bad for us but this is only because we have been brought up on foods that are far too sweet, with their appeal artificially enhanced by flavourings and colourants. Most food manufacturers have not the slightest interest in the effect of their goods on your body, merely on whether they have a pleasant taste and therefore will sell well. The immune system is no different from any other part of the body in requiring energy to function efficiently and it will not gain sufficient energy from 'junk' food. Furthermore there is plenty of scientific evidence to show that all these chemical additives have a direct depressant effect on the bodily defences.

One of my children recently had a friend to tea and we served up a plate of spaghetti bolognese which he refused to eat. On asking what sort of food he eats at home the reply was beefburgers, sausages and chips. Beefburgers and sausages are very often made with low quality meat disguised with flavourings and colourants. I was not surprised to hear that the child was absent from school the following week with a bad cold!

The general principle of healthy eating is that it is wholefood with no additives. There should also be a reasonable intake of carbohydrate and protein without excessive amounts of fat. Whenever I suggest this to parents it always evokes the reaction that this is impossible to achieve in children. This is partly because many people misunderstand the term 'wholefood', which simply means foods that have nothing added or taken away from them. They are not processed or refined and are near as possible to their natural state. Wholemeals are important as they contain the nutrients children need in a form they can use. A classic example of this is wholemeal bread, which is made from unrefined flour and contains natural wheat bran, which is a type of fibre. It is also packed with B vitamins and several minerals. To make white bread the flour is refined and in this process it loses most of these vitamins, minerals and fibre. My own son, Ross, used to eat slice after slice of fibreless white bread, whereas now he has switched to wholemeal and is satisfied after only one or two. A diet of refined foods results in children who are overfed and undernourished with a highly inefficient immune system.

Personally I find most books on diets, although describing excellent recipes, are not really designed for day to day living and are difficult to apply to children. So let us consider in practice how this can be approached. The two children we have followed in previous chapters, Simon and Julie, both had problems with their diets.

Simon's in particular was not at all healthy, starting with a sugar-coated breakfast cereal with full cream milk. Lunch was usually at school which was chips with everything and a fizzy drink. He would often have a packet of sweets on the way home and for tea would have a fry-up or a meat pie with tinned peas and baked beans. The deficiencies were fairly obvious and the changes reasonably easy. He liked porridge, which is a healthy start to the day and did not notice the change from full cream to semi-skimmed milk. Soon he came to enjoy a packed lunch for school especially when he could have the sandwiches of his choice as he loved mashed banana in brown bread. It is the main meal of the day that often creates the problems but if it needs to be prepared quickly then pasta is very simple. Even I can prepare a bolognese sauce to put on top which all my own kids love and I am sure it is true of most children. On evenings and weekends when there is more time, then a meat dish like chicken

	Original	**Change**
BREAKFAST	sugar-coated cereal plus full cream milk	porridge and semi-skimmed milk
LUNCH	beefburger and chips	brown bread sandwiches
DINNER	egg, bacon, sausages puddings	pasta and sauce yogurt/fresh fruit

Table 6.1: Typical changes in Simon's diet

Original	Change
tinned vegetables	fresh vegetables
tinned fruit	fresh fruit
sweets biscuits	chocolate
squash	fruit juice

Table 6.2: Typical changes in Julie's diet

served with potatoes and fresh vegetables is more nourishing than fried food. Children love yogurt, so either this or fresh fruit makes an excellent dessert. Table 6.1 summarizes the changes to Simon's diet.

Julie's diet was healthier than Simon's but the main faults were that it contained very little fresh food and she had a tendency to drink squash and eat sweets. There is a general principle that if you want to eat wholefoods then never open tins, as there are automatically additives in them. Sweets and squash are loaded with chemicals, all harmful to the immune system. Chocolate in moderation is much healthier. Such changes are shown in Table 6.2.

It is impossible to make all these changes at once, but if you introduce them gradually then your child will develop a much healthier immune system, which will then more easily fight off any tendency to asthma attacks.

Dietary Supplements

On one visit to the surgery Julie's father asked whether she needed to take anything in addition to her normal diet. I explained to him that vitamins are a group of substances which are essential for the life and well-being of our bodies; this particularly applies to the immune system. Growing children are very susceptible to vitamin deficiencies - only minute daily amounts are necessary but with the present method of preserving food these are often lost. Julie's father had read a little about vitamins in a library book but was confused by the vast number and obviously it is impossible to take supplements of all of them. As we are concerned in this book with preventing and treating asthma I will only mention the three vitamins that have been shown to help with this.

Vitamin A is found in milk, eggs and red vegetables such as carrots. The B vitamins, of which there are several, occur in wholegrain cereals, yeast and green leafy vegetables. Deficiency in both A and B reduces the production of the cells in the immune system which will fight off invaders before they have the opportunity to take hold. Vitamin C, which is found in fresh fruit and vegetables, is the third important supplement, as it specifically helps the immune system to kill invading viruses. The common cold, which often precedes an asthma attack, is particularly sensitive to increased doses of vitamin C. In addition it increases the ability to capture and destroy any other infections that actually gain a hold on the body. I recommended therefore to Julie's parents that she take regular daily supplements of vitamins A, B compound and C.

Exercise in Children

'Why can't we go in the car, Daddy?' If I hear this phrase from my children once more I shall scream! Our local supermarket is no more than half a mile away but always there is this inbuilt resistance to a simple ten minute walk. The immune system, like the rest of our body, thrives on exercise but scientific development seems determined to make our lifestyles become increasingly more sedentary. The motor car is the prime example but everywhere there are labour-saving devices. In shops there are lifts and escalators instead of stairs, airports have long walkways and at home there are electric carving knives and even power-driven toothbrushes!

If children are taught bad habits early in life they tend to persist into adulthood. In asthma there is no doubt that some kinds of exercise can bring on an attack but with the correct management this should not create any problem. There is also increasing evidence that the more exercise the child does take the less chance there is of wheezing developing. In other words the fitter the child the less asthma he or she will suffer. I am sure this is because of the increased efficiency of the immune system

I asked Julie and her parents how much exercise she was taking, and it turned out to be very little. She had only just started school, so her father always took her in the car as it was on his route to work and a friend's mother gave her a lift home.

I asked her about games at school: 'Well, we do have P.E. once a week in the school hall but we don't really do very much and I don't start netball until next year,' Julie replied.

This is quite typical of many primary schools these days and arises partly from lack of interest from the teachers but mainly from insufficient government funding for facilities and sports equipment. I also enquired about swimming but unfortunately Julie had been too late to enrol for lessons so only went occasionally. The main responsibility for her sedentary lifestyle, however, really lay with her parents who did not encourage her at all. In addition to not walking to school they never went into the country at weekends or took her to the local leisure centre themselves.

Simon also very rarely walked and although there was football and cross-country at school he found both of these tended to make him wheeze so he rarely put much effort into them. The end result of this lack of exercise is an unhealthy immune system and therefore little resistance to illness, including asthma.

Children love 'doing' things. They love exercising themselves as long as it is presented in an attractive form. While walking to the local shop may not hold much instant appeal I have found that my own children love walking up mountains! On telling them that to 'climb' Snowdon they would have to start training they immediately jumped at the opportunity to walk to school. All kids love swimming and it only requires a little effort to take them to the local pool once a week and the benefit to their body defences will be enormous.

Walking and swimming are the most beneficial forms of exercise and it is wise to start with them if your own child does not do anything else. Then, with the immune system strong it is easy to move on to sports like football, cross-country and cycling which put much more strain on the airways.

Stress in Children

It is now generally accepted, even in the most conventional medical circles, that stress in adults can precipitate illnesses. Recurrent minor afflictions often seem to occur when you are under the most pressure. Even more serious conditions like heart attacks and cancer can often be traced back to a major stressful event, of which a bereavement is the commonest. This tendency to illness is undoubtedly because of the depressant effect of stress on the body's immune system. This lowers our defences, allowing ill health to take over. Children, however, are just as liable to suffer from the effects of stress as adults and their immune systems are equally vulnerable. Obviously they do not have the same sorts of stress as their parents, as they are not concerned with balancing the housekeeping or wondering how to keep up with the mortgage payments.

Many specialists on asthma will maintain that it is the over-protective attitude of the parents that causes the tension in children which brings on an attack. It is natural, they claim, to do all you can to protect your child from environmental allergens, from catching cold and from the mockery of school fellows; but most parents take this too far and their child becomes very nervous and fearful of the slightest wheeze. To this I would say 'What a load of rubbish!' Obviously these so-called experts' own children have never suffered from asthma so they can only rely on theory and not on practical experience. My wife and I, like most parents I know, have never over-protected our own asthmatic children. In fact, we tend to do the opposite as we are keen that they should be able to lead normal active lives.

Certain children just seem more prone to suffer with stress in the same way that some adults do. Simon was a classic example, in that he was a natural worrier. At the age of 9 he would worry about practically anything but was at his worst at the end of school holidays. He liked school very much but for some strange reason a few days before the start of a new term would become very concerned, mainly at the thought of a new teacher. Once his parents realized this situation, they were able to reassure Simon that there was nothing to be worried about. This was in no way being over-protective. Stress in children is very common and can suppress the immune system in a very short period of time, perhaps taking only a day or two. An asthma attack can quickly follow. It is up to parents to recognize when their children are anxious or concerned and then to deal with this by massive reassurance. It is amazing that once their problems are shared then the stress is relieved and the immune system quickly recovers.

Just occasionally, stress in children persists even though the parents exert a calming influence. While tranquillizers are available I would very rarely recommend these and prefer to try a more natural approach. Sarah was a lovely 10 year old who was

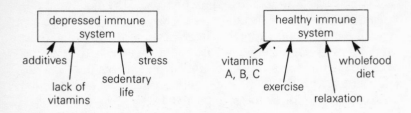

Figure 6.1   Factors affecting the immune system

very shy and used to worry continuously about going out to new places. Often trips out would have to be cancelled at the last minute when Sarah became wheezy. I suggested to her mother that we should teach Sarah the technique of self-hypnosis which would enable her to relax at times of stress. Her parents were very wary to start with at the thought of their young child being put 'under the influence'. However, they soon saw how effective it was as Sarah became much more settled. Not only that but it did her confidence a world of good to know she had an effective method of stopping her wheezing. I have discussed hypnosis and relaxation in more detail in Chapter 8.

I always think of the cells of the immune system as an army of soldiers who will march off to war against any enemy invaders. If these soldiers are kept in tip-top condition then they will be able to cope with virtually anything. Applied to asthma, all the viruses and allergens will not be able to gain a hold if the system is functioning efficiently. To do this it is necessary to boost it with a healthy diet, the correct supplements, regular exercise and as stress-free a life as possible. See Figure 6.1 which illustrates the factors affecting the immune system. Children like Julie are too young to be able to do this themselves and rely on their parents to help them. No parent wants to see their loved ones fighting for breath with asthma so you owe it to them to make the necessary changes in their lifestyle. You will be amazed how quickly and easily your child will take to them. If the immune system is kept strong you will go a long way to preventing any further asthma attacks.

CHAPTER 7

Avoiding the Causes

Preventing a wheezing attack by avoiding the precipitating causes may seem glaringly obvious but it is amazing how some parents choose to ignore this side of asthma control. A typical example was 10 year-old Ben, who was very allergic to his grandparents' dog and every time he visited them he developed breathing difficulties, which on two occasions were severe. I told his father firmly that either the visits must stop or the dog would have to go. He frowned at this suggestion and said he didn't want to upset his own parents! He had the choice really between removing the dog or possibly losing his own son. Now it is always upsetting to give away a family pet but it hardly compares with the life of one of your children. Happily the dog moved next door and Ben is able to visit his grandparents whenever he likes without the fear of an attack.

The irritable airways of the asthmatic child are influenced by a wide variety of triggers, and control can be exercised over some of them. Environmental temperature changes, fumes, fog and similar irritants can be avoided when possible. Infections can be reduced by avoiding close contact and psychological stresses can be anticipated. However, the main thrust of control is focused most sharply on the question of allergies and particularly the house-dust mite.

Both Simon and Julie, the two children we are following, suffer from some form of allergy - Simon has hay fever in the summer and Julie has allergic eczema - so it is reasonable to assume that allergies play an important part in the precipitation of their asthma attacks.

The House-Dust Mite

The main allergen to affect the airways is the house-dust mite. This is a small insect which is too small to be visible to the naked eye but can clearly be seen under the microscope. It is called the house-dust mite as it lives in and feeds off household dust. Since the mite congregates wherever there are warm humid conditions and flakes of human skin, it will predominate in bedrooms, mainly on mattresses, bedlinen and carpets. In an average bedroom many millions of these little bugs can be found and rather revoltingly it is their faeces to which sufferers are allergic. Both sets of parents looked disgusted when I told them!

I know my own children are particularly sensitive to dust, so we have to keep their bedrooms as clean as possible and I urged Julie's and Simon's parents to do likewise. The following steps are important and should be carried out regularly:

1. Use synthetic or cotton sheets and pillow cases. Do not have pillows that are filled with feathers. Both synthetic material and cotton are low allergy materials and house-dust mites don't thrive in them.
2. Wash the duvet every 2 or 3 weeks and the sheets and pillow cases every week.
3. The mattress should be enclosed in a plastic cover. As a high percentage of the mites will be in the mattress lining, this cover is probably the most important of all the steps against them. The alternative is to wash the mattress regularly but this is obviously not practical. Plastic covers are easy to fit and can be purchased at any of the large chain chemists. It might not seem very comfortable to sleep every night on plastic but it doesn't worry children at all.
4. Dust daily with a damp cloth on all surfaces.
5. All clothes and shoes should be put away in wardrobes and dressing gowns should not hang behind doors gathering dust.
6. Most books will recommend daily vacuuming of both mattress and carpet to remove the mites but if an ordinary vacuum cleaner is used then it can actually make the situation worse. The retaining mesh on a typical machine will not retain particles less than 8 microns in size. This means that the mites' faeces which are only 6 microns will be simply blown into the air, greatly increasing the allergic effect. The obvious

question if you don't vacuum is what about the mites in the carpet? Children, however, do not tend to lie on the bedroom floor with their faces buried in the shag-pile so they will not inhale the allergens from the mites. Only if the carpet is vacuumed and the mites are showered into the air will problems then arise. Anyone who is really worried about the bedroom carpet can always replace it with wood flooring or linoleum but I personally have never found this to be really necessary and it is certainly less comfortable.

By following these steps the allergic effect of the house-dust mite can be greatly reduced.

Change of Climate

Julie's parents raised the serious question as to whether they should consider moving house to a different area or even a new country. In only a very few instances would 'yes' ever be the answer to this question. Evidence to support this solution is largely circumstantial. Old damp houses near rivers or the sea do contain more house-dust mites, whereas dry centrally-heated houses contain less. Damp houses do harbour moulds which can also produce allergens, making an asthma attack more likely.

No area should really be considered right or wrong for asthmatics as some seem to improve with one set of environmental conditions and others from another. The only really proven benefit of moving is if you go to the clearer air of a country like Switzerland. Davos is well known for its asthma clinics and it claims that the benefit to chest sufferers is that the atmosphere is unpolluted. Recent research has shown, however, that it is probably simply that the house-dust mite does not like high altitude so does not exist in the mountains of Switzerland. I therefore reassured Julie parents that they did not have to move house, and if they followed the steps in this book her asthma would be well controlled anyway!

Animals

Simon's father was worried as to whether he should take action against the family cat. In Ben's case at the start of this chapter it was obvious that the grandparents' dog was the cause of the wheezing, but in the majority of children the role of animals is less clear-cut. So how can you tell if the family cat, dog, guinea-pig, parrot or whatever is to blame? It is only in very few instances that an animal allergy is the only cause for asthma and often it is only one among many. Before making any decision that would cause distress, some sort of trial separation must be arranged. While holidays away from home are the most convenient way they are not ideal as the lack of the family pet is only one of many environmental changes that take place. It is preferable to arrange for the animal to be put into a cattery or kennels while the child stays at home and every other facet of the home environment is kept constant. Particles of animal hair and dander will lie around the house for some time in household dust so that separation will need to be accompanied by a thorough cleaning programme. If there is a dramatic improvement in the asthma then it is reasonable to assume that the pet is the major precipitating cause. In my experience, however, if the animal allergy is only one amongst several triggers, then removal of the animal is unlikely to be of great benefit.

Food Allergy

During her infancy Julie had suffered quite badly with cracked dry skin, a condition called atopic eczema, and her mother had read that this can be caused by an allergy to milk. Does this then play any part in her asthma? There is no doubt that for a proportion of children with asthma, allergic reactions to foodstuffs are important as a cause of their condition. As I mentioned in Chapter 3 the foods most commonly incriminated are cow's milk, eggs, wheat, cheese, yeast, fish, pork and peanuts. Some children are sensitive to the preservatives or colouring agents used by food manufacturers and in particular tartrazine and quinoline in squashes and cola. While it is often difficult to identify the aggravating foodstuffs it is worth eliminating each one in turn from the child's diet to see if there is improvement.

Atopic or allergic eczema as in Julie's case is indeed associated with a milk allergy. This could be strongly suspected by a careful history of her progress through infancy and by seeing if she had suffered any of the following symptoms:

- Colic
- Irritability
- Repeated vomiting
- Diarrhoea
- Snuffly nose
- Chestiness
- Poor sleep pattern
- Persistent nappy rash

Taken in isolation many babies have one of these symptoms, but if your child has at least three of these then a milk allergy is a strong possibility. Julie, in fact had suffered from all of them at different times and her mother kept her off milk for six weeks. During this time Julie seemed much happier and livelier without any sign of wheezing. It was reasonable to assume therefore that milk allergy was certainly playing a part in her asthma.

Both Simon's and Julie's parents asked about desensitizing injections. This arose with particular reference to the house-dust mite, as although it is possible to keep the bedrooms clear of dust in their own houses what would happen when they went to stay with friends and relatives or were away on holiday? In these circumstances the rooms would not be free of the dreaded mite and consequently breakthrough asthma could well occur. In an attempt to overcome these sorts of problems researchers developed a method of stimulating the body's defence system to produce more of the cells which cope with individual allergens. Unfortunately, this method, although having the potential for curing asthma, has two major drawbacks.

First, the stimulating solution has to be given by a series of injections which are administered once a week for eighteen weeks and repeated each year for three years. Secondly, it is unusual in asthma for there only to be one allergic cause. We have already seen that Julie is allergic to both house dust and milk and no doubt there are others, so there seems little point in desensitizing her to only one of these. Mixing two or more allergens in the one treatment always brings disappointing results as it seems the immune system can only deal with one allergy at a time.

Consequently I never now recommend desensitization as it is cruel, if not barbaric, to subject a child to weekly injections. If there was a guarantee they would work then a case could perhaps be made, but not otherwise. Both Julie's and Simon's families

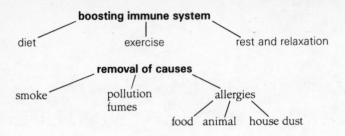

Figure 7.1   Treatment plan

seemed relieved when I rejected the desensitization approach.
Figure 7.1 shows the stages we have covered so far in our treatment plan.

CHAPTER 8

Prevention Using Complementary Medicine

No one likes the idea of taking drugs on a long-term basis, and because of this many people are turning to complementary - or alternative - medicine to provide a different approach. The thought of giving your own children regular daily medication is equally disturbing and parents usually ask if there is any way this can be avoided. Personally, I am a great advocate of non-drug therapy and will recommend a suitable course of treatment whenever possible. The only proviso I have is this: asthma is a serious condition, and conventional medicine can offer every child virtually complete freedom from attacks using a sensible and logical treatment plan as outlined in this book. You should certainly think twice before varying from this plan as this is a decision taken on behalf of your child which he or she has no power to understand or refuse.

My advice is to use alternative methods only for prevention and for mild asthma attacks. When a child has a severe wheeze this is potentially dangerous and it is vital to use a method of treatment that is guaranteed to work. If the breathing is very distressed I would always stabilize the condition using conventional medication first as outlined in the chapters on treatment. This is mainly because natural methods do tend to be more gradual in onset and speed is vital when the asthma is severe.

When your child has been free of a wheeze for some time then it would be safe to introduce an alternative therapy with careful reductions of the drugs. If this can be undertaken with the help of your doctor then so much the better, although I know full well that many GPs still have very rigid and old-fashioned views about anything at variance with their own narrow training.

If used in this way then there are several non-drug therapies that are excellent and certainly worth trying. Simon, the 10 year old we have been following, always had a problem with his asthma in the few days before returning to school. His mother also commented that as soon as an attack starts he becomes very frightened and upset. This anxiety is very common in all children with asthma, and relieving it would go halfway to allowing them to lead a normal life.

Relaxation

Any approach to this anxiety must centre on relaxation. The fear aroused by the approach or the actual experience of an attack of asthma causes tension. This can be felt in the muscles around the neck, the shoulders and the chest. It is also likely that it is reflected in the muscles around the airways and this is why increasing tension does escalate the distress produced by an attack. Being aware of tension is the first step to relieving it. Each muscle group can be taught to be tensed and then deliberately relaxed and techniques that are learnt when the asthma is quiet can be brought into use when wheezing starts.

'How on earth can I teach a 10 year old to relax?' asked Simon's mother when I suggested this. It is surprising how easy it is to achieve this in children and how receptive they are to this approach. In Simon's case you could see the tension in his posture, as the tightening of his shoulder and neck was making him round-shouldered and hunched up, so his chest muscles were being constricted. I taught him to relax these areas and allow his posture to revert back to normal. Suddenly from a rather nervous looking boy he was standing tall and erect and looked generally more confident. On subsequent occasions as soon as his wheezing started Simon was able to unhunch his neck and shoulder muscles thus allowing his chest to fully expand. The most sophisticated use of relaxation and muscle control is in yoga and older children - particularly teenagers - can easily practise this either at home or at a local class.

Most people think of the term relaxation in relation to calming the mind, and this is a very important aspect of asthma control. Some doctors even go as far as prescribing tranquillizers - which is totally wrong in my opinion - but it does confirm the point that remaining relaxed is vital. Deep relaxation of the mind really merges in with self-hypnosis, so I will describe these together a little later in this chapter (see p. 61).

Breathing Exercises

Beyond simple muscle relaxation comes the question of breathing exercises, which are usually taught by a physiotherapist. One of the major factors in asthma is tightening airway muscles, and if these can be relaxed then the affect is highly beneficial. Unfortunately these muscles are not under direct voluntary control; however, by regulating the aspects of lung function that are controllable there is no doubt that the muscles in the airways will relax. These controllable aspects include the rate and depth of breathing combined with other muscle groups which move the chest.

Deliberate alteration in the frequency with which breaths are taken is one of the more obvious ways in which control can be exercised over breathing. In asthma the airways are narrowed, so it is obvious that more effort is required to force air in and out through a narrow tube than to blow gently and gradually through a wider one. It takes less effort to breathe slowly and deeply through narrowed airways than it does to breathe rapidly and shallowly. Some children with asthma find they adopt this pattern naturally but most - usually from panic - seem to breathe more quickly than is really necessary. This soon makes them distressed, so the important message is to inhale slowly followed by gentle breathing out.

There is no doubt that relaxation and slow breathing are proven scientifically to be beneficial. Controversy surrounds the various techniques which claim to move one part of the chest more than another. The muscles involved in breathing fall into three groups: the diaphragm, which is at the base of the lungs; the muscles between the ribs; and the muscles around the neck. It is the diaphragm which really holds the key to controlled breathing in children with asthma. This is a dome-shaped muscle situated beneath the lungs which is attached to the trunk all around its outer edge. When the muscle fibres in the diaphragm contract during breathing in, the whole dome of the diaphragm moves downwards towards the abdomen drawing the lungs with it. This, in effect, expands the lungs, allowing more air to be taken into them.

When a child has an asthma attack there is automatic tightening of the muscles of the upper abdomen, and this prevents the downward movement of the diaphragm. The description 'diaphragmatic breathing' is given to techniques whereby this movement of the diaphragm is synchronized with relaxation of the abdominal wall. However, this breathing is not really diaphragmatic but abdominal.

The technique is difficult to teach to young children and it did not play a significant part in Julie and Simon's management. However, many parents reading this book will have older children who will be able to control their breathing very easily. It is well worth a visit to a local physiotherapist to be properly taught the technique. It can, however, be learnt at home by following these simple steps:

● As you breathe in, as well as allowing your chest wall to expand, ensure that your stomach is filling out. This relaxes the stomach muscles and allows the diaphragm to move downwards.
● On the breath out, concentrate on deflating your stomach with a slow gentle movement.

In other words you are working at using the stomach to breathe rather than the chest. Of course the chest will really be doing most of the work, but this is automatic, whereas using the stomach is not. Learning this method of breathing will ensure that the correct pattern is maintained when wheezing develops, and help the attack to be better controlled.

Alexander Technique

This is a technique for helping certain conditions including childhood asthma. It is taught by physiotherapists as well as specialist Alexander teachers, so it seems appropriate to consider it at this point. It was developed by Frederick Matthias Alexander and the theory states that a great deal of illness can be traced to the way in which we use our bodies; muscles are tense when they should be relaxed, backs are humped, vertebrae are contracted together, the neck is sunk into the chest, legs are constantly crossed and toes turned in, tensing and straining all the muscles and joints of the body. These tensions greatly contribute to many of the complaints in contemporary society, including arthritis, back pain, rheumatism and fibrositis. If there is poor posture of the upper body it leads to hunching of the shoulders and poor chest expansion. If a child's lungs are unable to expand fully this can tip the balance and send the child into an asthma attack.

Certainly in Simon's case there was marked room for improvement in posture, as he was very hunched and generally did not stand straight. The Alexander Principle propounds that in the conditions of modern life we have lost the natural use of our bodies, often taking on in very early childhood bad habits of posture and movement copied from our elders. These habits are so ingrained that when we are shown the correct use of our bodies it seems 'wrong' to us. The Alexander method therefore involves a course of retraining and in my experience children are far more receptive than adults.

Alexander himself was an asthmatic and developed his method by experimenting in front of a mirror. He had received very little help from doctors but noticed that by stopping certain muscular tensions in his neck and chest his breathing was greatly improved. He discovered that the way he was using the rest of his body was also affecting the way he worked generally.

The Alexander method is really a demanding approach to personal living which can lead to a personal freedom and health but it requires a willingness to work on oneself. I asked my practice physiotherapist to work on Simon, who is now standing straight and has much fuller lung expansion. He already looks far more self confident and all this will greatly help his asthma.

Hypnosis

There is no doubt that when Simon's asthma attack started he became very frightened, and this fear greatly worsened the degree of wheezing. Under these conditions it is often difficult to achieve adequate relaxation, especially if the child is young. The perfect solution would be for Simon to go to sleep, but this is not usually possible in any child until the attack starts to improve.

I explained to Simon's parents that a much deeper form of relaxation is hypnosis. Naturally they appeared wary - the history of hypnosis is very chequered, as it has been practised by charlatans, frauds and tricksters. The situation is very different today and hypnosis is rapidly gaining respectability and is widely used in many medical conditions. The state of hypnosis is basically a changed level of awareness or consciousness somewhere between being fully awake and asleep. It is a level which is very pleasant and extremely relaxing.

Most people when they are asked if they have ever been hypnotized will answer 'no', but they are nearly always mistaken. Almost everyone has at some time been in a hypnotic state without recognizing it. Childhood day-dreaming – often so real to the child that the imagined situation takes the place of ordinary reality – is essentially self-hypnosis. In adult life a common example is when driving down a familiar road you may suddenly realize that you have travelled several miles without being able to remember anything of that part of the journey. If you have a passenger at the time he or she would be able to testify that you had driven perfectly competently.

Theatrical acts often show hypnosis in an amusing light, when people appear to be made to do all kinds of weird things either against their will or certainly out of character. This is actually an illusion, as there is no way anyone can be hypnotized if they don't want to be and similarly no one can be made to say or do things which are offensive or wrong. Furthermore, as in the driving example above, you can always come out of the hypnotic state at any time, so there is never the situation as on stage where a character is wandering round in a trance waiting for someone to say the magic word to release them! It is common to be aware of noises from outside the room or simple sensations like shoes being too tight, but these seem somehow distant or removed. Hypnosis does not involve losing or giving up control. The experience is under your control and yours alone, and the process can teach a degree of control over mind and body that is not there for most of us in the ordinary waking state. It is in fact one of the most relaxing, pleasant and comfortable experiences you can have.

Once the basic hypnotic state is achieved it is then possible to learn the technique of self-hypnosis, so that you can put yourself 'under'. Simon's parents were convinced about the possible benefits of hypnosis but they still couldn't understand how it could be performed on a child or how they could learn it themselves.

They brought Simon into the surgery and I settled him into a comfortable chair, allowing his parents to remain at the back of the room. Laying a hand on his shoulder I asked him to close his eyes and imagine he was playing on his favourite beach. Slowly, by asking him to take deep breaths, Simon became more and more relaxed until he reached a state of hypnosis. I was then able to make him feel so happy that his breathing became calm and rhythmical.

With Simon so relaxed his mind was in a very receptive mood, and I then focused his thoughts solely on his asthma, suggesting that much of his problem lay in being a worrier. A typical example was that his attacks were precipitated by returning to school. If he could become calmer and less anxious then his tendency to wheeze would disappear. As well as relaxation it is also possible under hypnosis to induce positive thinking and this I did with Simon by asking him to repeat five times: 'I am not going to have any more asthma attacks and my breathing is going to stay normal.'

There is no doubt that if positive suggestions are repeatedly made to your brain - especially under hypnosis - beneficial effects will eventually start to happen. However, it does take some time for this to occur, and since it would have been impractical for Simon to come for treatment every day, self-hypnosis was the obvious answer. While he was still under hypnosis I suggested to him that he should lie on his bed the following day, close his eyes and count five deep breaths in and out. At the end of the fifth one he would be very relaxed and in a state of hypnosis. He would then repeat the phrase about his breathing five times and then relax for ten minutes. At the end of that time by counting slowly to seven Simon would return to normal consciousness. I don't think his parents thought for a moment that their energetic, lively son would ever discipline himself to carry out this procedure every day. However, it is amazing how well children take to hypnosis - much more readily than adults - and I am sure this is because they do not have the reservations or the inhibitions of their elders.

I saw Simon a week later and he certainly was very bright and cheerful. He had practised self-hypnosis every evening and had obviously impressed his school chums, although his attempts to put them into a trance had not been successful! Over the subsequent months he has learnt to take himself deeper and deeper into his subconscious which has enabled him to focus his thoughts specifically on his asthma.

In my opinion the age of 10 is the perfect time to learn hypnosis and it is a technique which will prove useful throughout later life. I myself often use it to relax for five minutes during a busy surgery to enable me to clear my mind fully for the next patient. Unfortunately, for a 4 year old like Julie, relaxation techniques including hypnosis are difficult - though not impossible in patient and skilled hands. However, other alternative methods - in particular homoeopathy which is described below - are particularly suitable for little ones and I would have no hesitation in trying this out in Julie's situation.

As this country is obsessed with drug-orientated medicine, there are very few doctors practising hypnosis under the N.H.S. However, outside the medical profession there are very many people offering hypnotherapy for a wide range of conditions, from blushing to stammering. Many of these practitioners are skilled in what they do but unfortunately there are always a few who have not had adequate training. Altering the workings of the human mind is complex and I for one would wish to know that the person who was using such techniques on my own children had the right qualifications and was known to be good at his or her job. I would urge anyone who wants their asthmatic child to try hypnosis that they find either a doctor or clinical psychologist to do this. Fortunately attitudes are changing and nearly all GPs will be able to recommend a suitable one.

Homoeopathy

Of all the alternative methods that have been tried in the prevention of asthma, homoeopathy is the one I favour the most. It is completely safe, has proved remarkably effective in my own children and I have used it with excellent results on many of my younger patients.

Unfortunately, as with any specialist skill there are some rogues about who are not adequately trained in the subject. In my experience, if homoeopathy sometimes seems inadequate it is mainly because the wrong preparation is prescribed rather than the child being unsuitable for homoeopathic treatment. The only drawback is that the preparations do take time to work and therefore are not suitable for treating an acute attack of asthma. Some homoeopaths will recommend homoeopathic treatment for every aspect of asthma, which in my opinion can be downright dangerous; for a severe wheezing episode it is vital to stick to well-tried conventional drug therapy which we know will be effective.

Homoeopathy is a system of medicine that was discovered in the early 1800s by a German doctor who had become dis-illusioned with medicine, with good reason. At that time, physicians believed that sickness was caused by humours or fluids that had to be expelled from the body by every possible means. To achieve this end patients were cauterized, blistered, purged and bled. Not only that but it was customary to mix any prescribed medicines together. In fact one of the 'cures' contained more than fifty ingredients. This German doctor, named Hahnemann, was quickly denounced by his colleagues and enraged chemists, who were as powerful as our drug companies are today. No doubt he would have been similarly ostracized by contemporary doctors.

The principle of homoeopathy is that 'Like is cured by Like'. This means that a remedy can cure a disease if it produces in a healthy person symptoms similar to those of the disease. This preparation can be given in a very dilute form, so it doesn't actually cause the symptoms but is sufficient to produce a cure. This can be a difficult principle to understand; I always find it much easier to follow if it is likened to a vaccine.

Take for example Simon's immunization against measles; the vaccine contained a minute dose of actual measles, injected into Simon's body through his skin. This dose was not sufficient to cause him to become ill and show the symptoms of measles but was enough to trigger a reaction in his immune system to fight off this condition. If at any time Simon should be exposed to the measles virus in the future, then his body would immediately produce the same defensive reaction again. So it is in homoeopathy; taking asthma as an example, a small amount of a substance which causes wheezing is given to the child. This then produces a massive reaction in the immune system to fight off the asthma. By giving homoeopathic tablets regularly this immune system is kept in a constant state of defence against an asthma attack developing.

The choice of remedy is vital, and one of the features of homoeopathy is that diagnosis considers the person as a whole being. In other words, although asthma is a condition affecting the lungs it is also a reflection of the child's emotional and mental make-up.

Everyone with asthma is wheezy, but there are many individual variations so I have prepared a checklist to make it easier to match the child's symptoms to the remedy:

1. Colour of skin: pale or red?
2. Colour of lips: red or pale? Dry or cracked?

3. Colour of tongue: red-tipped, red-streaked, white, or swollen? Is it dry or wet?
4. Expression: frightened, confused or calm? Do the eyelids droop?
5. Movement: is the child quiet and still, lethargic or restless?
6. Mood: irritable, nervous, angry or sad?
7. Skin: dry, moist, clammy, hot or cold?
8. Voice: weak, hoarse, deep or husky?
9. Speech: incoherent, rushed, slow or does the child refuse to say anything?
10. Smell: sick, sour, musty or offensive?
11. Physical needs: is there a craving for fresh air? Are hot or cold drinks asked for and does the child like to be rubbed with a cold or warm flannel?
12. Time of day: does the wheezing tend to occur in the morning, afternoon, evening or is it worse at night?

This list sounds complicated but only takes a minute or two to work through. In each individual child, although the asthma attacks vary in severity, the features are nearly always the same. Once the remedy is chosen, it can therefore be taken time and again.

There are four principal remedies that can be used to prevent wheezing:

- *Arsenicum Album*. Suitable for use when the following symptoms are apparent: red skin, red lips, red moist tongue, frightened, restless although quickly exhausted, nervous, moist hot skin, weak voice, rushed speech, sickly smell, worse after midnight. There is a craving for hot drinks and a dislike of the cold.

- *Carbo Vegetabilis*. Suitable in a child whose attacks are characterized by: bluish skin, pale lips, pale dry tongue, intense fear, quiet and weak, sweaty skin which is cold and clammy, hoarse voice, very little speech, sour smell to breath, worse in the evenings. The child feels better away from heat and likes a cold flannel.

- *Ipecacuanha*. Pale skin, pink lips, clean dry tongue, calm and not frightened, cold sweaty skin, normal voice and quite chatty, smells normal, worse in the night and morning. Likes cold weather and cold drinks.

- *Nux Vomica*. Red skin, red lips, red dry tongue, irritable and impatient, weak husky voice, skin very sensitive to touch and feels hot, smells bitter and is worse in the morning. Vomiting is a major feature during an attack and the child likes warmth and rest.

You will notice that the features of each preparation are easily distinguishable. Your own child may well not show every one of these characteristics, and the closest-fit remedy should be chosen.

Let us now apply them to our two children. Simon's parents had noticed that he was always very flushed during an attack, and was frightened. Exhaustion was rapid and he spoke with a weak voice. The attacks came at night and he always wanted a hot drink in a warm place. He was ideally suited therefore to the preparation *Arsenicum Album*. Julie was really quite the opposite, in that she tended to have a bluish discoloration to her skin, lips and tongue, with cold clammy skin. On that first attack she had been intensely afraid and had spoken in a hoarse voice. Her mother had soothed her with a cold flannel and Julie didn't like the gas fire on. *Carbo Vegetabilis* would be the treatment of choice in her situation.

Homoeopathy is emerging as a vigorous alternative to standard medicine, and an increasing number of physicians are now practising it. Members of the royal family have been treated in this way for over two hundred years. It is safe and cheap and is becoming increasingly available on the National Health Service. So if your child is struggling with wheezing episodes and you would like to try a non-drug method of treatment, do not be afraid to ask your own GP to recommend a suitable homoeopath in your area.

Acupuncture

When I first learnt about the technique of acupuncture, the thought of sticking needles into children seemed a horrible idea. Over the years, however, I have come to realize that it is almost a painless procedure, and that children are far less afraid of it than adults. Its beneficial effect in the prevention of asthma is well documented, although why this occurs is not absolutely proven. Julie's mother had found relief following a course of acupuncture for a painful back, so was most interested when I suggested it might be used in her daughter's situation. Acupuncture originates from China and is used there routinely in all medical conditions.

While I don't fully accept all the theories of Chinese medicine, as one Chinese teacher once said to me, it is not necessary fully to understand the workings of the engine of a car in order to drive it. Similarly it is not vital to understand completely how acupuncture works in order to practise it. Chinese medicine is based on the idea that the body functions by taking energy out of the air. This enters either through the hands or feet and is distributed to the different organs of the body through a system of channels rather like a railway network. There are six channels in each arm and six in each foot, making twenty-four in all. These channels follow a tortuous course up the limbs supplying energy to the parts they pass through before all ending up in the brain. An example of these channels is shown in Figure 8.1,

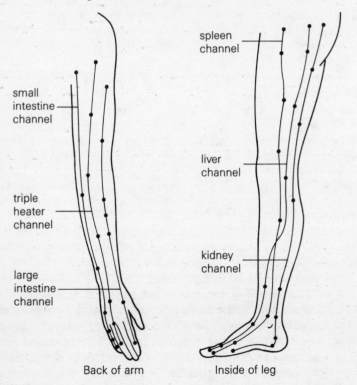

Figure 8.1   Acupuncture channels and acupuncture points

using the back of the arm and the inside of the leg as illustrations.

If the energy flow down the channels is easy and uninterrupted, then the organs supplied with this force will remain in perfect working order. Supposing, however, one of the channels becomes damaged, then the flow of energy will be interrupted and problems will arise. In asthma it is the flow down the lung channel that is affected and this shows itself by the development of wheezing and shortness of breath.

It follows that if this flow of energy can be restored then the wheezing can be stopped and normal lung function will resume. This is achieved by inserting acupuncture needles into the relevant channel, at different places. These places are called acupuncture points, and have been mapped out over the years by practitioners of acupuncture. If these needles are then stimulated, either by gentle twisting or by a low frequency electric current, then energy will pass into the channel and the obstruction will be overcome.

Certainly Julie, being only 4, was a challenge, but she turned out to be remarkably co-operative. The needles are very thin and very sharp so they are hardly felt as they pass through the skin. They differ from needles used for injections which are much thicker as they need a channel through them to inject the liquid. In fact, Julie did not feel the needles at all – the main problem was keeping her still. Treatment was concentrated on the lung channel, which starts in the hand. The first needle was inserted as near to the commencement of the channel as possible and in this case near to the base of the thumb. I have found through experience that it is rarely necessary to use more than four needles at a time. Some acupuncturists use a dozen or more but this seems unreasonable to the patient and raises doubts in the therapist's belief in the treatment. So Julie had four needles in her hand and arm and these were stimulated gently with a mild electric current for fifteen minutes. During this time Julie's mother read a book to her to keep her quiet and still. I repeated this treatment weekly for four weeks and at each appointment I listened to Julie's lungs and checked her peak flow readings. Over this time she became much calmer and her lungs became clearer, giving her more energy. I now see her every few months for a reinforcing dose but generally she has taken to this method of treatment very well and has never been deterred by the needles.

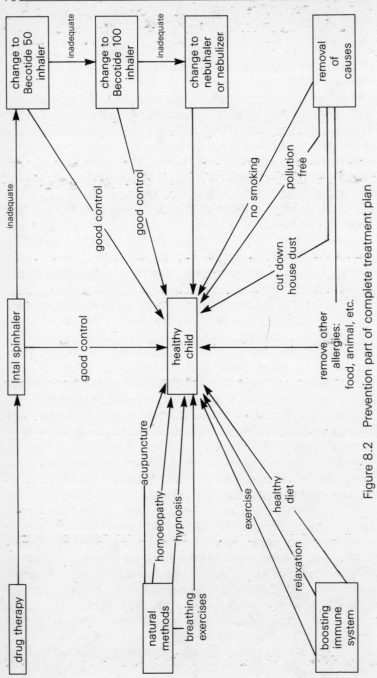

Figure 8.2   Prevention part of complete treatment plan

This is not true of all children however, and 10 year-old Simon would not even consider them. If the children are afraid and cannot be reassured then acupuncture is doomed to failure, as relaxation is impossible and the needles will not enter the channels correctly.

I can certainly recommend consideration of acupuncture as a preventive technique if you are against continuous drug therapy or to enhance the effect of the medication. Its major disadvantage is that it takes a considerable amount of time, as each session lasts about half an hour and is given weekly at the outset. It is also vitally important to go to a suitably qualified therapist, as at the present time anyone who wants can set up as an acupuncturist. Your own GP should be able to recommend a suitable one.

I have discussed the various alternative methods of asthma prevention in some detail in this chapter as there is so much interest in non-drug therapy these days. To recap, there are basically four methods: breathing exercises; relaxation with or without hypnosis; homoeopathy; and acupuncture. There are others, including herbal medicine, aromatherapy, colour therapy or reflexology, but these are less proven and I am wary of suggesting these on account of the potential severity of the condition. I must confess that with asthma being a potentially life-threatening condition I always recommend initial control with inhalers in all but minor attacks, and only when this has been achieved can the inhalers be slowly reduced by adding an alternative method of prevention. The choice depends very much on personal preference.

We have now reached the end of the section of this book on prevention of asthma and Figure 8.2 shows the completed step-by-step plan to stop attacks occurring.

Treatment of Asthma Attacks

CHAPTER 9

General Treatment of Asthma Attacks

An acute asthma attack implies that the child has become increasingly short of breath with a marked wheeze and the combination is causing increasing distress. So far in this book I have discussed the various methods of preventing this happening, and so I hope you never need to utilize the following section on treatment. Unfortunately, the nature of the condition does mean that most asthmatic children will at some time have at least one significant attack, and for some they may be recurrent.

An acute attack is very frightening for both parents and child and it is vital therefore to have an effective plan of treatment which you know will work. Your own calmness and lack of panic will then give your child reassurance and confidence, and the attack will settle much faster. If the wheezing does not improve rapidly then there can be only two possible explanations. Either the medications are not being taken correctly, or your doctor has prescribed the wrong one. By using the treatment plan in this book you will at least know that the choice of drugs is correct. In the next chapter I will describe fully the method of taking the various types of medication available, and I would certainly recommend every parent to study this at a time when their child is well.

There are basically two changes during an asthma attack. Firstly the muscles in the airways tighten up or go into spasm, so it is difficult to breathe in sufficient oxygen with each breath. Secondly the lining of the breathing tubes becomes swollen, causing further narrowing. It is logical therefore that treatment should be aimed at relieving both these factors.

Bronchodilators

As the spasm precedes the swelling, most initial treatment is aimed at the former. The group of substances used for this purpose are known as bronchodilators, and the large measure of success achieved in the control of asthma attacks centres on these remedies. A daunting array of products has been produced, mostly for commercial reasons, but I have found that there are two - namely Ventolin and Bricanyl - that are most effective and, as they have been used for many years, are known to be safe.

The dilemma with bronchodilators is by which route they should be administered. All of them are most effective when injected, but this is neither desirable nor practical. For general use there are only two reasonable ways - by mouth or by inhalation.

Since most drugs in this country are given by mouth there is a time-honoured custom in favour of this route. There is one major drawback - as the drug has to pass all round the body to reach the lungs, large doses must be taken. Bronchodilators which are inhaled pass directly to the organ in trouble, and so are not absorbed into the rest of the system. Taking Ventolin as an example; one inhalation contains 100 micrograms of the drug, whereas one tablet contains two milligrams - twenty times the dose of the inhalation. Thus, the potential for side-effects is many times greater with tablets. In my own practice - except in children under the age of two who are too little to master an inhaler - I never now use oral bronchodilator therapy. This is partly due to the possible unwanted effects, but also because their action is so much slower and often speed of treatment can be vital during an attack.

The main drawback with inhaled bronchodilators is that, because the airways are narrowed, insufficient of the drug may actually pass into the lungs, although this only really occurs when the wheezing is very severe. The most popular way of giving either Ventolin or Bricanyl is by pressurized inhalers. A jet of the drug is released by pressing the cannister into its plastic casing. To inhale the drug the cannister must be triggered just as a breath in is being taken. Some children find this difficult and therefore the treatment will be ineffective. Drug companies have tried various methods to overcome this problem and have devised a type of inhaler where a capsule is inserted full of powder and this is then inhaled. This comes in two forms, either as a rotohaler or as a diskhaler; this is similar to the way Intal was inhaled for the prevention of an attack.

More recently two new forms of inhaler have been produced which are proving very useful. Firstly, there is an Aerolin autohaler, which is similar to the pressurized inhalers but is breath-activated, so does not require precise co-ordination of pressing the base of the inhaler as you breathe in. The drawbacks are that if your child is very wheezy the reduced force of inhalation may not be sufficient to trigger the device. Secondly, there is the Bricanyl turbohaler, which, like the autohaler, is breath-activated but a powder is inhaled and not a spray. It also has the same drawback of needing sufficient force of inhalation to fire it. However, both the autohaler and the turbohaler have removed the problem of co-ordinating the pressing of the inhaler with the breath in and for this reason have become my first choice in treatment.

Pressurized inhalers, however, are by far the commonest in use so I will concentrate on these. The pressurized inhalers, the turbohaler and the autohaler can all be carried easily in pockets and taken to school without the worry of breaking open capsules and whether the powder is dry or damp. One of the major reasons for worsening of an asthma attack is poor inhaler technique, but I have found that nearly all children can learn the correct method if sufficient time is taken to teach them. At my own surgery we run an asthma clinic and much of each appointment is taken up in teaching the correct technique for these inhalers.

Just occasionally a child may find it impossible to co-ordinate their breathing while pressing the cannister so there are some 'tricks of the trade' to overcome this situation. First, Bricanyl can have a plastic tube fitted to the end of it, known as a spacer. Instead of the puffed drug going straight into the mouth it first fills this tube and can then be inhaled into the lungs. Both Ventolin and Bricanyl can be first squirted into a large plastic container called a volumatic and then be inhaled more slowly over several breaths. The disadvantage of this method is that the containers are large and cumbersome so cannot be carried in the pocket.

If the attack is severe, and the child too distressed to use the inhalers properly, or if the bronchial tubes are so narrow that the powder will not reach the lungs, then a new technique involving a nebulizer can be used. A measured dose in liquid form is poured into a small container and this solution is then vapourized using an electric current. The child inhales the vapour via a mouthpiece or facemask over a period of ten minutes.

The nebulizer is very effective and has completely changed the outlook of severe attacks, as now nearly all children can be managed at home and do not need the trauma of hospital admission. These nebulizers are inexpensive and every home with an asthmatic child should have one. It may be the best buy you ever make.

As the success of treatment is so dependent on the technique of using the different inhalers and the nebulizer, I have devoted Chapter 10 purely to learning the correct method. I can only urge everyone to spend some time mastering them. It is now possible to obtain dummy inhalers from your doctor so you can practise without inhaling an actual drug.

Steroids

As well as using bronchodilators it may also be necessary to reduce the swelling of the airway linings. The only effective method is to use steroids, which are usually given in the form of cortisone. Many parents gasp when I suggest this, but in actual fact when given over a short period of time they do not have any harmful side-effects. Taken in inhaler form, like Ventolin or Bricanyl, they will never cause unwanted effects. If administered as tablets it takes over six weeks of continuous usage before the child runs into problems; usually only a five-day course is needed. The steroid inhaler I would recommend is Becotide, which is made in differing strengths dependent on the child's age and severity of the asthma. They also make a solution for use in the nebulizer. By having the right medication available and by using the correct technique, I am confident that everyone who follows the treatment plan will quickly be able to settle their child's attacks.

Basic Medication to Have at Home

- Ventolin or Bricanyl inhaler
- Ventolin or Bricanyl nebulizer solution

- Becotide inhaler
- Becotide nebulizer solution
- Prednisolone (Cortisone) tablets

A rotahaler or diskhaler can be used as an alternative to an ordinary inhaler.

For babies Ventolin or Bricanyl medicine may be necessary.

CHAPTER 10

Inhaler Technique

It is estimated that about 55 per cent of children do not use their inhalers correctly. This means that not only do they not obtain the full benefit from them, but it is much more likely that a serious or even life-threatening attack will develop. Sometimes the inhalers may even be discarded as useless.

Simon was a classic example. He was given a Ventolin inhaler, and when his technique was checked at our asthma clinic a month later, he was pressing the cannister when he was breathing out and all the drug was being blown into the atmosphere.

By using the following steps the maximum benefit can be obtained:

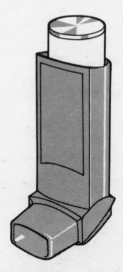

Figure 10.1 Simple pressurized inhaler

A Pressurized Inhaler (see Figure 10.1)

1. Remove the mouthpiece cover.
2. Shake the inhaler vigorously before use.
3. Hold the inhaler upright and breathe out as far as possible.
4. Place the mouthpiece in your mouth between your teeth and close your lips firmly round it without biting.
5. Just after starting to breathe in through your mouth, press down on top of the inhaler to release the medication while still breathing in steadily and deeply.
6. Hold your breath, take the inhaler from your mouth and continue holding your breath for as long as is comfortable. This is vital because if you blow out too quickly the drug will not be retained long enough in the lungs to be effective.
7. If you are to take a second dose, then wait about fifteen to twenty seconds before repeatings steps 2-6.
8. After use always replace the mouthpiece to keep out dust and fluff.

It is important not to rush this procedure, and if you see a mist coming from the top of the inhaler then you are either not breathing in deep enough or are pressing the inhaler at the wrong moment. A little practice will soon correct this problem.

An Aerolin Autohaler (See Figure 10.2)

1. Remove the mouthpiece cover.
2. Shake the inhaler vigorously.
3. Place the mouthpiece in your mouth between your teeth without biting.
4. Take a deep breath in. This will release a measured dose into your mouth.
5. Hold your breath for as long as possible.

You will see this is identical to the pressurized inhalers except that it is breath-activated, and so does not need to be pressed as a breath in is taken.

A Turbohaler (see Figure 10.3)

1. Shake the inhaler vigorously.

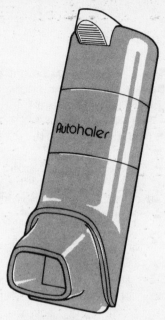

Figure 10.2 Autohaler

2. Twist the bottom of the inhaler first one way and then back again.

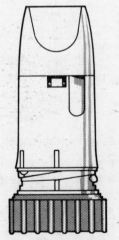

Figure 10.3 Turbohaler

3. Place the mouthpiece in your mouth without biting it.

4. Take a deep breath in, and as the device is breath-activated a measured dose of powder will be inhaled into the lungs.
5. Hold your breath for as long as possible.

A Rotahaler (see Figure 10.4)

1. Ensure that the capsules are dry.
2. Push the capsule into the special slot in the bottom of the rotahaler.
3. Twist the middle of the rotahaler forwards and backwards. This slices the capsule in half, releasing the powder.
4. Place the mouthpiece in your mouth between your teeth and close your lips round it without biting.
5. Take deep, strong sucks so the powder enters the lungs.
6. Remove the old capsule and shake out any little bits of powder remaining.

Again it is important not to rush the procedure. Two deep sucks should be sufficient if the technique is correct. If it takes more than this, then an incorrect method is being used. Try not to let your child suck and blow alternatively as this will make the capsules damp with saliva.

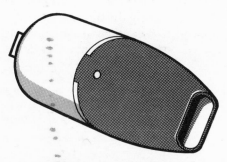

Figure 10.4 Rotahaler

A Diskhaler (see Figure 10.5)

(a) Loading the device

1. Remove the mouthpiece cover and ensure the mouthpiece is clean.
2. Hold the corners of the white tray and pull out gently until the

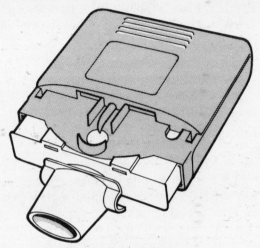

Figure 10.5 Diskhaler

ridged areas on the sides of the tray are fully visible.
3. Squeeze the ridged areas and pull the tray, with the wheel, out from the diskhaler body.
4. Do not remove the wheel. Place the disk on the wheel with numbers uppermost and then slide the tray back fully into the body of the diskhaler.
5. Rotate the disk by moving the tray out and in gently, until the number 8 appears in the indicator hole. As the device is used this indicator hole shows the number of doses remaining.

(b) Using the device

1. Hold the diskhaler firmly in a level position. Lift the rear edge of the lid and raise it as far as it will go until it is fully upright, thus puncturing the blister. Some resistance will be felt as the upper and especially the lower surfaces of the blister are pierced.
2. Close the lid.
3. Keeping the inhaler level, breathe out fully.
4. Raise the diskhaler to the mouth and gently place the mouthpiece between the lips without biting. Do not cover the air inlets on either side of the mouthpiece.
5. Breathe in through your mouth as quickly and as deeply as you can.
6. Hold your breath briefly to allow the powder to reach the

lungs and then remove the diskhaler from your mouth.
7. Slide the tray out and in once so that the next number appears in the indicator hole. Do no pierce the blister until immediately before inhalation.

Each disk consists of eight blisters containing medication. When the number 8 reappears in the indicator hole, all eight doses have been taken and the disk should be replaced by repeating the procedure above. Please make sure you do not throw the wheel away with the empty disk. All this sounds very complicated but in practice is simple and does have the advantage over the pressurized inhalers of not requiring co-ordination of breathing in while pressing the cannister. The major disadvantage is that as each disk only contains eight doses it is necessary to carry spare disks and often children forget. I have also found they do tend to clog up with powder. The manufacturers do provide a brush in the rear of the diskhaler body to clean any remaining powder. This should be carried out with the tray and wheel removed from the body of the diskhaler but again in my experience children cannot be bothered to do this, and the efficiency of the device is gradually reduced.

A Volumatic

(See Figure 5.6 page 41.)

1. Place the standard pressurized inhaler into the end of the volumatic as shown in the diagram.
2. Put the mouthpiece between your teeth and close your lips without biting.
3. Press the end of the inhaler twice so that the medication is squirted into the volumatic.
4. Take four or five deep breaths in, pausing between each one to allow the drug to pass into the lungs.
5. Remove the pressurized inhaler from the volumatic and replace the cap to keep the mouthpiece clean.

This procedure should be done calmly and slowly. The major advantage is that it is not necessary to co-ordinate breathing in with pressing the inhaler. Also it is possible, when necessary, to increase the dose by pressing the inhaler more than twice. It is quite safe to give up to five puffs at any one time, or more if recommended by your doctor.

A Nebulizer

(See Figure 10.6.)

1. All parts should be thoroughly cleaned before use.
2. The reservoir should be filled with a standard dose from either a Ventolin or Becotide nebule or a Bricanyl respule, depending on which your doctor has prescribed.
3. As in the diagram, one end of the plastic tube is connected to the nebulizer and the other end to the bottom of the reservoir. The mouth piece or mask is then connected to the top of the reservoir.
4. The nebulizer is switched on and the spray that is produced is then inhaled with normal breaths. This is carried out for ten minutes by the clock.
5. All parts should then be washed clean before the machine is used again.

The nebulizer, while usually electrically operated, is also available in footpump form, where the power is generated by regular pumping. This makes it considerably cheaper, and useful for holidays and travelling. The disadvantage is that it is very tiring pumping continually for ten minutes, so an electric machine is preferable for routine use.

As a final point, please do not listen to well-meaning but misguided friends or relations who will say that inhalers and nebulizers are dangerous or toxic. In truth they are very safe, extremely effective and however much you give it is difficult to overdose with them.

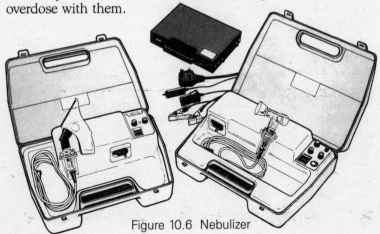

Figure 10.6 Nebulizer

Treatment of a Mild Attack

Asthma attacks can be mild – an irritating cough or wheeze but the child is not ill – or they can be more severe, causing increasing shortness of breath. The mild and severe attacks do seem to be two separate conditions, with a mild attack not necessarily leading on to a severe one. The management of each is different, so I have accorded each a separate chapter.

David is an 8 year old who has gradually developed asthma since the age of 5. His parents noticed he would occasionally wake in the night with a slight wheeze, which also occurred when he climbed hills. (During the sleeping hours the airways do close down a little, so any tendency to develop asthma is accentuated at night.)

Pressurized aerosols which can be carried around with the child are very much the best treatment for mild attacks. Initially I had prescribed David a Ventolin inhaler, but he had some problems co-ordinating his breathing, so I switched him to a Bricanyl turbohaler. This produced a dramatic improvement and quickly relieved his wheezing with a single puff. I loaned him a peak flow meter to try and discover the severity of the condition. David's normal peak flow reading was 400.

I asked him to repeat this the next time he became wheezy, and one morning the following week he woke up with an irritating cough and slight shortness of breath. This time when blowing into the machine the counter only reached 310, a 23 per cent reduction in his breathing capacity; this was sufficient to cause him to cough and have a slight wheeze. He repeated the reading two minutes after a slowly breathed in puff on his inhaler, and the reading had risen to 375; his breathing felt completely normal at this level. When he showed me these results at his next visit to the asthma clinic I decided to be a perfectionist and advised David to try two puffs instead of one. This extra dose returned his peak flow reading to 400, his usual healthy level.

The use of a bronchodilator inhaler in this way is the simplest form of treatment, other than sitting down and resting. It is all that many asthmatics ever need, to them the inhaler can be their best friend. I had told David's parents when I saw them on their own one day that they must not give him the impression that they were very worried about his attacks; if they behaved as if these mild wheezing episodes were almost a part of normal everyday living, then David himself would not become stressed or frightened by them. This is a very important part of managing asthma – and as it transpired David never picked up any of the emotional traumas of asthma at all.

In the majority of cases, therefore, the therapy for a mild asthma attack is very straightforward – two or three puffs on a pressurized bronchodilator inhaler and a check on the peak flow meter that the lung capacity has returned to normal. Unfortunately, there are occasions when treatment may not be that easy – even for very mild attacks – so it is worth looking at some other cases to see the different situations that arise.

Let us take the case of Julie, who we have been following throughout this book. When I first started treating Julie for asthma she was only 4, and at this age it does take a little longer to master the technique of using the inhalers. Her asthma had first presented with a particularly severe attack, and her parents were worried about this happening again. It appeared on closer questioning that Julie had been having minor wheezing episodes about every 10 days, so I started her on an Intal spinhaler, which is used to prevent any attacks developing. (This device is described in detail in Chapter 5, p. 35). A capsule is inserted and punctured by sliding the base of the spinhaler. The powder in the capsule is then inhaled.

While Intal is effective at reducing the frequency of asthma attacks, it is still possible to suffer with wheezing – especially in Julie's case when she had a cold. I tried her with a standard pressurized Ventolin inhaler which she didn't like and couldn't co-ordinate breathing in with pressing the cannister. In fact most of the dose was lost in a cloud of vapour down her nose! Julie thought this was horrid and I realized quite quickly that if I didn't try a different method I would soon lose the willing co-operation of my patient! Furthermore, using the pressurized inhaler hadn't made the slightest difference to her peak flow readings. Julie had a special junior model and her readings were normally exactly 250, reduced to around 200 when she became wheezy. On repeating this after the pressurized inhaler the readings did not alter, indicating that none of the medication was reaching her lungs.

As she was well practised in the use of a spinhaler it seemed a logical step to try Julie on a rotahaler, since this also involved the use of a capsule. This meant that she did not have to co-ordinate the breathing in with any other action, and all it required was two slow, deep inhalations to breathe in the powder. On re-checking her peak flow levels after treatment I found they had returned to their normal level of 250. The rotahaler comes in a compact little box which also carries six rotacaps. I stressed both to Julie and her parents that it was essential to make sure that the rotacaps were replaced when used. Several times I have heard of children who come to use their rotahaler only to find they have no spare capsules.

Julie's parents asked me at what stage she should start to use her rotahaler, and whether she should continue her Intal spinhaler as well. It is a cardinal rule in asthma that the earlier an attack is treated the quicker it will settle. I therefore advised them to give her a rotacap as soon as they suspected a wheeze to be starting. This can then be repeated every three hours if necessary. As Intal is designed to prevent attacks developing, once wheezing is established there is little point in continuing it, so it should be left alone until the asthma has subsided.

One of the most important aspects of the treatment of asthma is that the child should have faith in the treatment and be certain that it will relieve them. I always ask the girl or boy what their thoughts are about the particular type of inhaler they are using, as sometimes it throws up unexpected reactions. Julie's comment about the pressurized inhaler was mainly about its taste and not the fact that it came down her nose! Also she liked the taste of the powder in the rotacaps which was surprising because to me it tastes foul! In fact Julie was very happy with her treatment, as the rotacap was easy to use and it was something to show off to her new school mates.

I asked Simon, the other child we have been following throughout this book, to describe to me how he felt during an asthma attack:

I always seem to get them before I go back to school – or at least my Mum and Dad say I do. I remember waking up in the night and I suddenly found I was itching. At first I didn't know what was making me itchy but suddenly I noticed a lot of white and red spots all over my body. When I was itching I really caught one and it hurt a lot. I felt very hot as if I was in a train boiler. I felt very weak and tired and then I started to cough. I couldn't stop and my Mum came in and shouted, 'Stop that coughing, you'll waken everyone else.' I tried to hold my breath so as I wouldn't cough but I found that my breathing was worse than usual. I needed the toilet but when I got out of bed and tried to walk I found I couldn't breathe. I felt very depressed and started to cry. My Mum came then and said that I was having an asthma attack and needed my inhaler. I took two puffs of my inhaler and soon I felt a lot better although my hands wouldn't stop shaking. I couldn't sleep so my Mum stayed with me the rest of the night.

This describes one of Simon's early attacks, and now he is well able to recognize when his wheezing is going to start. At the time I was treating him with a standard Ventolin pressurized inhaler, which was effective at relieving the wheezing but gave Simon the irritating side-effect of shaking characteristic of Ventolin. His parents were very worried by it, so I changed him to a Bricanyl inhaler. Next time I saw him at the asthma clinic he commented that the Bricanyl made him seem very weak and he always had to lie down after it. He had also found that if he used it at school he was unable to concentrate on his lessons. I had not heard of this previously with Bricanyl so wondered if it was really a facet of the asthma rather than the treatment. However, at his next appointment Simon still complained of tiredness and said he much preferred the shaking with the Ventolin - it only bothered his parents, not him. Often in illnesses children seem to know naturally what is right for them, so I changed Simon back to the Ventolin. Although he developed the shakes again he was quite happy and not tired or lethargic.

Simon was a classic example of how important it is to monitor asthma with a peak flow meter. When he was perfectly well and had been free of any wheezing for a few weeks his peak flow measurement was around the 450 mark. When I saw him after school one day when he had developed asthma following a run, his peak flow was down to 330, indicating a reasonable degree of constriction of the airways. Ten minutes after taking two puffs on his inhaler it had risen to 390. Simon was very happy with this and felt much better, but really he still had some way to go to a full return to normal.

I checked Simon's inhaler technique and there was no doubt he was rushing the process and not allowing the medication sufficient time to be absorbed into his lungs before breathing out. I told him to breathe slower and this time his peak flow rose to 420, better, but still 30 short of his maximum.

One of Simon's friends at school had shown him his diskhaler, which Simon thought looked good fun and I then wondered if inhaling a powder would improve his peak flow. Sure enough, with one single measured dose, roughly equivalent to the two puffs he had been taking, the peak flow reading returned to its normal of 450. Simon went away very pleased with his new toy and looking forward to showing it off at school.

Only by measuring Simon's peak flow could we tell that his lungs were not functioning normally. I cannot stress enough the use of the peak flow meter in the treatment of both mild and severe asthma, as it shows quite objectively whether the situation is improving or becoming worse. As the child becomes older the readings can be used to gain valuable time in treatment and also to assess how severe the attack is likely to be.

Sarah was a 14 year-old who became very skilled at using the peak flow meter. She commented, 'I found that a great reduction in my peak flow would usually occur and only produce a mild wheeze initially. However, if I didn't take action at that stage to correct the wheeze then my breathing would become more and more difficult.' In other words her peak flow fell faster than her wheeze developed, but the wheeze would eventually catch up. She adds: 'I often referred to my peak flow meter as my early warning system. Since starting at the asthma clinic I have been in the habit of recording peak flow at the same time each morning and evening. While I use Intal as my preventive medication, as soon as my readings show any fall I switch to my pressurized Ventolin inhaler. I have been able to catch attacks at an early stage and stop my breathing becoming too bad.'

It is interesting to speculate as to why peak flow should be a better indicator of airway obstruction than one's own awareness of breathlessness. I am sure the answer is that unless you have to run or climb stairs you can suffer quite a large diminution in your respiratory efficiency without being fully aware of it. If you are in good health then it is difficult to realize what an enormous difference there is in your requirements for oxygen when walking on the flat compared to going upstairs or running. Asthmatic children soon become particularly aware of this discrepancy but, even so, can be deceived. When lying in bed or sitting still, little oxygen is needed and it is easy to be misled as to how difficult it may be to breathe in more oxygen when required.

Sarah agreed with this observation: 'I have found that my normal peak flow rate is 480, but this can fall to about 350 at rest and I will not feel breathless. As soon as I start to move about, though, I notice that I cannot breathe. Sometimes in bed at night I have woken up and felt my asthma has subsided only to find when I get out of bed to go to the toilet that I am far more breathless than I thought.'

A good analogy is with the weather: a fall in barometric pressure is a warning sign of rain to come. One final point at this stage on peak flow: it is usual for the readings at night to be automatically some 50 points lower than the morning level. The reason for this is not understood, but it suggests that perhaps the airways in some ways narrow at night as less air is required.

So far we have controlled a mild asthma attack with a bronchodilator, either taken via a pressurized inhaler or as powder from a diskhaler or rotahaler. We have seen how the requirement and effect of these can be accurately assessed with regular peak flow readings.

Equally important in the treatment of an attack are supportive measures. Simon the 10 year-old always became very frightened when his wheeze started, in case his attack became severe. The inability to breathe is in itself a frightening and horrible experience which provokes considerable anxiety. (In fact, the mechanical interference with respiration has been used for many years as a method of torture. People being interrogated have their heads plunged underwater until they nearly drown; victims have slabs of stone piled on the chest until it becomes more and more difficult to breathe.) Anxiety actually increases difficulty in breathing, so it is vital that it is controlled. Fear and worry make the breathing more rapid and shallow, and it is exactly the opposite which is required during an attack.

Simon was taught to breathe deeply and slowly, and I stressed to his parents the importance of encouraging this when wheezing is present. One difficulty with deep breathing is that it tends to bring on a cough, and coughing at the height of an attack makes the wheeze worse. With experience, however, the child will learn to breathe just deep enough to prevent the cough occurring.

In past years many children had oxygen cylinders in their bedroom, but this had little therapeutic value unless the attack was severe enough to be life threatening. Too much oxygen can actually depress the respiration further.

The anxiety which accompanies difficulty in breathing is also relieved by the presence of a loved one. Simon always wanted his mother to be with him, as he found being able to hold her hand was enormously comforting. No asthmatic needs telling that breathing is easier when sitting up, and most children will have their preferred position. This may be propped up in bed with several pillows, or when wheezing it may be easier to breathe if the legs are hanging downwards, so sitting in a chair - providing the child can keep warm - is usually more comfortable. The idea that one must be in bed if ill is a difficult notion to dispel in many parents, but there is no doubt asthma is better managed in an armchair downstairs.

Both Simon's and Julie's parents asked me whether they should encourage their children to eat during an attack. For some reason the appetite disappears entirely when wheezing, but it is important to take in sufficient calories to provide energy. This should be little and often - perhaps as a biscuit or piece of chocolate where the energy will be quickly available to the body. As well as eating it is necessary to drink as much fluid as possible, unless this causes vomiting. I find that lemon barley is well tolerated by most children and is better than simple tap water, often so heavily chlorinated it tastes unpleasant. The effort of trying to breathe can lead to dehydration and there is some evidence that the extreme stickiness of the sputum or phlegm is reduced if sufficient fluid is taken.

Sleep is always a problem, and I have found at home that the first night of an attack is usually spent downstairs in front of the video recorder. It is much better now that we have all-night television but in the old days when there was no night entertainment the morning often seemed a long time coming. It is important that children with asthma should not be woken for any reason once they have fallen asleep. The audible wheeze always sounds much worse when asleep, but if the breathing deteriorates further it will always make the child wake up anyway. The benefits of going to sleep are very great, as not only does it produce relaxation but also reduces the body's energy requirements. For this reason I sometimes prescribe a gentle sedative to help induce sleep.

These steps that I have outlined above will settle nearly all mild attacks of asthma without recourse to further measures. However, there are a few children where the response to bronchodilator inhalers is less than would be expected. To understand the reason for this we must look again at why the wheeze occurs. Spasm or contraction of the muscles in the walls of the airways is undoubtedly the initial problem but there is also the swelling of the lining of the breathing tubes to take into account. Some children undoubtedly develop much more swelling than others and this can prolong the breathing difficulty. Bronchodilator inhalers will relieve the muscle spasm but will not ease the swollen linings.

Debbie was a classic example of this, as although her initial wheeze improved with her bronchodilator inhaler she was left with a persistent cough and some shortness of breath. This was not relieved by increasing either the frequency of the dose or the number of puffs she took. The most effective treatment is to use a cortisone inhaler in which a measured dose of steroid is taken directly into the lungs. Please do not be doubtful about the use of cortisone as insufficient is absorbed into the rest of the body to cause any unwanted effects.

Debbie's parents asked what exactly steroids are? 'Steroid' is a name given to a group of chemical compounds, many of which occur naturally in the body. There are a wide variety with different effects. For example, there are the muscle-building steroids used by some athletes illegally to improve their performance. There are also steroids in contraceptive pills and steroid creams for the treatment of sore, inflamed skin. Cortisone is used in asthma as it is a very powerful anti-inflammatory agent so will relieve the swelling in the affected airways. The preparation I recommend is Becotide and this is available in all the same devices as Ventolin and Bricanyl – a pressurized inhaler, a diskhaler or a rotahaler. Debbie was used to the simple pressurized inhaler, so I prescribed Becotide in a similar form. The dose was two puffs four times daily which we were able to stop after four days when her peak flow had returned to normal. It is important to note that the swelling of the airway lining does not settle anywhere near as dramatically as the spasm, so it may take some time for the child to return fully to normal.

On one occasion when Debbie used a steroid inhaler she

noticed her voice became a little husky, and she developed a mild throat infection. This can sometimes happen, but neither effect is serious and both can be prevented or reduced if the mouth is rinsed out after using the inhaler. Should it continue to be a problem then using a spacer device like a volumatic (a chamber into which the inhaler is puffed) will also cut down the problem, by reducing the amount of the drug which lands in the mouth and throat.

One of the potential difficulties of a steroid inhaler is that it is most needed when the linings of the airways are already swollen. When this occurs much more phlegm than normal is produced. This is usually quickly dried up by the inhaled steroid but occasionally there is so much phlegm that the steroid spray is unable to penetrate through it, and instead of quickly clearing the attack there seems to be very little effect. One answer, as in the case of 9 year-old Alison, was simply to increase the strength of the inhaler. She was already using an inhaler called Becotide 50 which released 50 micrograms of steroid at each puff. By changing her to Becotide 100, in which 100 micrograms are released, there was enough penetrative power to dry up the phlegm and restore the airway linings to normal.

In adults it is possible to increase even further the strength of inhaler, to one called Becloforte. I would not recommend this in children, as recent studies have shown that at this high dosage there is significant absorption into the rest of the body, and so there is potential for troublesome side-effects.

My own son Ross is typical of a small group of children who, although their wheezing is controlled, always have a trouble-some cough, especially at night. Serial peak flow readings never quite reach normal. Ross was taking both a Ventolin and Becotide 100 inhaler, but there was still a suggestion of some low-grade swelling of the airway lining. On account of this I decided to try giving Ross his therapy via a nebulizer for a few days. Basically he received the same drugs, but in a more inhalable form. The nebulizer is an electric machine which passes a stream of air through a special solution of either Becotide or Ventolin. This is turned into a vapour which is inhaled either via a face mask or mouthpiece. The nebulizer is mainly used for severe attacks, so I have described it in more detail in the next chapter, but it can also be used in mild attacks that do not fully clear.

In practice I stopped both Ross's pressurized inhalers and

substituted the nebulizer on a three times a day basis. The nebulizer drug solution comes in specially prepared ampoules which are squirted directly into the reservoir in the nebulizer, thus ensuring the correct dose is given. The machine is switched on and the vapour inhaled for ten minutes. As Ross was not ill he was able to watch television when this was happening. In actual fact he did not require the Becotide as well and within two days his peak flow was back to normal and that irritating cough had vanished. It would have been quite alright to have used Becotide as well but it is often not necessary. The main drawback to using both drugs is they cannot be mixed together in the nebulizer, so it takes a full twenty minutes for each treatment session. This does not matter if children are ill but when they are well it produces intense fidgeting and lack of co-operation!

Babies and Children Under the Age of Two

Very young children present a special problem when they are wheezy, as they are too young to use any of the conventional inhalers. Many doctors will not recommend them until the age of 3, but I have found with care and patience most children will manage with them quite adequately from the age of 2 onwards. The situation has improved since research has shown there is no possibility of overdosage, as people always feared. In fact the nebulizers have been shown to deliver up to 50 times the dosage of a conventional pressurized inhaler.

Asthma is uncommon below the age of one, and the reason for this is uncertain. It seems likely that it does take some time for irritability of the airways to develop, and perhaps there is some inherited protection from the mother in the first year of life.

If a baby does develop wheezing it is usually mild and often requires no treatment. However, if it becomes more severe then it may be necessary to give a bronchodilator, either Bricanyl or Ventolin in a syrup form by mouth. This obviously raises the possibility of side-effects, but in babies the dose needed to produce widening of the airways is very small, so it is unlikely that significant unwanted effects will arise. The main problem with medicines at this age is they are very slow to act and may take over an hour to produce any effect at all.

An alternative to medicine - especially in the 1-2 age group -

is to use a conventional pressurized inhaler with an inverted paper or plastic cup on the end. Paul was 13 months when he had his first significant wheezing attack. It was not surprising, as both his parents suffered with it and were well versed in the use of the various inhalers. I advised them to give Paul some Ventolin every three hours using the following method. Firstly, a hole should be cut in the bottom of the plastic cup, big enough to fit the mouthpiece of an inhaler. The wide part of the cup is then placed over Paul's face and nose and four puffs of the inhaler are given into the cup. This manoeuvre allows the spray to stay in the cup long enough to be inhaled a little at a time with each breath without much effort. Paul received instant benefit and his breathing became much more settled.

Alternatively, Ventolin can be given via a nebulizer as described on p. 86. The problem with this method in the very young is that they will not tolerate a mask strapped to the face or a mouthpiece in the mouth. However, it is usually possible to hold the mask near enough to the baby's face for sufficient of the vapour to be inhaled. You will actually be able to see the baby breathing in the cloud of medication as it comes out of the nebulizer. This can be repeated as necessary, but four hourly is usually adequate. It is worth mentioning here that babies do tend to wheeze for longer than older children, although it often does not cause them any distress. Many is the time in the surgery where I have seen a baby with a slight wheeze who was nevertheless perfectly happy, and it was the parents who wanted something done. With some babies it is wise to allow the wheeze to settle on its own. This is not true, of course, in older children where it is important to bring the wheeze under control as quickly as possible.

I am normally a little reluctant to recommend alternative methods in treating asthma, as it is a condition which can deteriorate so rapidly. However, in young babies asthma is much milder and often responds well to homoeopathy. By using this it may well be possible to avoid the use of conventional medicine by mouth.

Homoeopathy treats the whole person, and so it depends a great deal on character and personality as to which preparation is most suitable. Basically I use four different types for the treatment of an acute attack:

- *Arsenicum Album.* When the baby is very restless though appears exhausted. The wheeze is usually worse between midnight and two in the morning. The baby is thirsty but will only take small sips of warm fluid.

● *Ipecacuanha*. The baby is vomiting or obviously nauseous and has a loud rattly cough.

● *Kali Carbonicum*. Attacks typically occur later in the night, usually between three and five in the morning.

● *Aconite*. Attacks usually occur after exposure to a cold wind and the baby looks very frightened.

Of all these I tend to find that *Ipecacuanha* is the one I nearly always prescribe, and if you are in doubt I would suggest trying this first. Homoeopathic remedies are available on prescription, but many GPs will not prescribe them. Fortunately they are very cheap and all of the above can easily be obtained from any health food shop. Although they come in tablet form they are not to be swallowed, but must be allowed to dissolve in the mouth. This is a great advantage in babies, anyway, since there can be a danger of choking with swallowed pills.

In this chapter I have described the treatment of a mild attack; by following these steps you will find your child's asthma will settle. It may seem complicated on first reading, but in reality it is very simple and straightforward. Please do take the obvious precautions like always ensuring that your child has his inhaler with him and that it is not empty. A standard pressurized inhaler contains two hundred doses, and although it is impossible to tell accurately how many remain a new one does feel much heavier than an empty one. So when an inhaler seems to be becoming very light make sure you have a spare one, and do not leave it until it is empty before contacting your doctor. In fact it is much safer to have at least one spare inhaler at all times and I know in my own house there are several in different places. For example my own child has one in his bedroom, one at his grandmother's, another in his trouser pocket and finally a spare one at school! Most GPs are quite happy to give an initial stock of inhalers to the child to ensure they do not run out. Another irritating problem about inhalers is that even a relatively full one can simply stop working.

The powder-containing inhalers – the rotahaler and the diskhaler – obviously have the advantage that there is no guesswork involved about remaining doses. However, it is still necessary to carry around spare disks or capsules and it is amazing how many children I have come across walking around with an empty rotahaler or diskhaler.

In the main children take very well to inhalers and certainly prefer them to tablets and medicine. One 8 year-old called Kirsty commented:

> When I had asthma once my dad had broken his arm and it was Christmas time. I felt very tight in my chest and all dizzy and sick. All I could manage to eat was soup and it felt like I was on a diet - especially as everyone else was tucking into Christmas food. Mum started to give me tablets to make my chest better but I hated the taste of them so I hid them around my room. Later when she tidied up my room when I was better, she found them all over the place! She shouted at me saying, 'I've found another . . . and another . . . and another . . .!' I just went downstairs and laughed to myself.

There are many special situations relating to asthma attacks - during exercise and when on holiday for example - but I have dealt with all these in Chapter 13 for ease of reference. Remember, if you can treat your child's asthma with confidence then the attack will settle quickly; you can start to gain that confidence by following the chart shown in Figure 11.1.

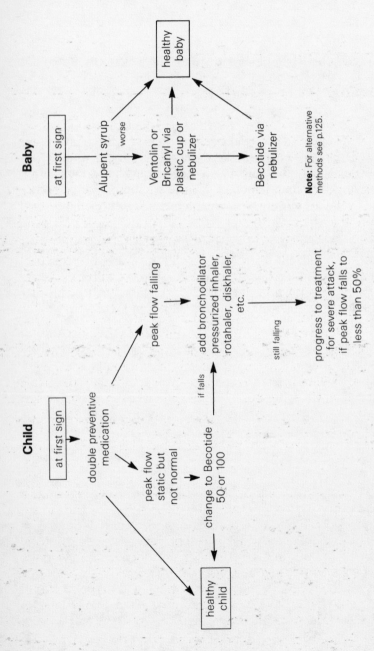

Figure 11.1   Treatment of mild attack

CHAPTER 12

Treatment of a Severe Attack

This is the time when asthma really hurts, when as parents you experience the pain and torment of seeing your own child suffering terribly in a desperate attempt to breathe. This is the time when an all-consuming panic can set in. You will be well aware that a certain number of children die every year from asthma, and suddenly you realize that your own son or daughter could be one of them. Surely it cannot be happening. Why can it not be like any other Sunday night? Why is it always at a time when the surgery is closed? You will feel desperately lonely and very frightened. 'Why did I not listen to what the doctor told me and give the inhaler three times a day as advised? I daren't ring again as I have already rung twice this week and it is a Sunday night.'

All these emotions and more will flash through your mind, and you will try to stay in control as you know that if you panic your child will sense this, and this can make the asthma worse. I know this is what happens as I have experienced these feelings myself with my own children. Perhaps as a doctor I should be better able to deal with the situation but I can assure you it is impossible for anyone to remain detached about their own family!

I remember on one occasion we had just returned from a holiday in Abersoch in Wales, and my son Ross had developed an attack of asthma in the car on the journey home. North Wales does not have that many hospitals, and anyway it wasn't until the last half an hour that his condition deteriorated rapidly. I rang my own GP and she came over immediately. Ross by this time was worn out with the effort of breathing, and in the middle of his nebulizer treatment he actually slumped into a kind of exhausted sleep and the mouthpiece fell out of his mouth on to the floor. At that moment I glanced at the doctor and saw a look of terror in her eyes – I knew for an instant she thought he had died. Fortunately Ross jerked himself awake and carried on with the treatment but I vowed from that day on that I would always be available to parents if they were struggling with their child's asthma. It was following that incident I opened an asthma clinic at my surgery, with no appointment needed, so anyone who wanted could come in at any time.

But what if it is at a weekend or when the surgery is closed? When should you call your doctor out? There are specific indications when to do this which I outline in more detail on p. 109. As a general rule you must always contact your GP if you are worried. Do not be concerned about contacting him or her unnecessarily. All doctors know that asthma is a potentially serious condition and that the sooner it is treated the better. Unfortunately there will always be the occasional doctor who will be a bit grumpy and might even infer that the visit was not needed. My advice to you if this happens is to immediately change your doctor to one who is more sympathetic. The vast majority will come out quite willingly even when it is in the middle of the night.

What does irritate doctors is to be called to see little Johnny at three in the morning when he has been ill for two weeks with a cold, or when the call has been left until one in the morning when the parents have returned after a night out!

Two years ago one of my asthmatic patients called Robert, who at that time was 14 years old was asked to write an essay at school on the subject of illness. He chose to write about an asthma attack he had experienced a few weeks previously.

I woke up totally unable to breathe. I was in bed, panting away, concentrating totally on how I could get enough air into my lungs. I was not in control of my breathing as this had become totally automatic and I had not been able to slow it down. I realized this was the worst attack I had ever had and the worst I had ever heard of. I was unable to get out of bed and did not have the breath to shout my parents. After another few minutes the attack had shown no signs of subsiding, I suddenly realized that I was in danger. I remember thinking to myself if this goes on much longer I am going to die. I prayed for God to help me and pull me through. At that moment I seemed to become detached from my body and was looking down from the ceiling. It was almost as if someone was telling me I would be alright if I managed to get to my nebulizer. At that moment my mother came in, as she had heard me cry out, and gave me my machine. I quickly recovered and always have the machine at my bedside now in case it happens again.

This description shows how important it is to know the correct treatment to give for a severe attack of asthma. The child is often in a very distressed state and as a parent coherent thought is very difficult. In this chapter I have outlined in straightforward terms the steps to be taken and the summary chart at the end can act as a quick reference in times of trouble.

Treating a mild attack of asthma is easy because there is no tension or stress involved and there is time to consider the best course of action. There are definite indicators to tell you when your child's condition is worsening and you should take stronger measures to control the attack. The following are the guidelines that I have found to be reliable:

Early Signs
1. No relief is obtained from the usual inhalers.
2. Your child requests more frequent doses of the inhalers.
3. There is a persistent wheeze which seems to be worsening.

Later Signs
1. Constant loud wheeze.
2. Child becoming easily tired.
3. Usual inhalers needed every hour.
4. Marked movement of the abdomen with every breath.

Danger Signals
1. Wheeze lessens due to shallow breathing.
2. Child exhausted.
3. Blue tinge to the lips.
4. Child very restless.

A more accurate guideline is the peak flow meter. As I have described on p. 37, this is a small device which is used daily to monitor the progress of asthma by measuring the amount of air which passes through the lungs. Any reduction in the score from the normal, healthy range will reflect a deterioration in the asthma. I would suggest that you use the following principles as a guide to the severity of the attack, using a score of 400 as the norm:

1. A score in the region of 300 to 400, i.e. a reduction of up to 25 per cent of normal, is classed as a mild attack and can easily be managed by the steps outlined in Chapter 11.
2. A score between 200 and 300, i.e. a reduction of up to 50 per cent of normal, is a sign that a serious attack may well be building up. You should not put off taking remedial action in the hope that the asthma will improve by itself – usually it does not.
3. Any score of less than 200, i.e. less than 50 per cent of normal, means the asthma is not controlled and has moved into the severe attack range. It should not be accepted under any circumstances and steps must be taken urgently to correct it.
4. A score of 100 or less, i.e. a reduction of 75 per cent or more, requires urgent medical attention. While it may be acceptable to try and see whether the treatment described for a severe attack is effective, you must only try this while waiting for the doctor to arrive. If your GP is unable to call within 30 minutes then your child should be taken to the nearest casualty department. I must stress, however, that this is a most uncommon occurrence and most probably the peak flow

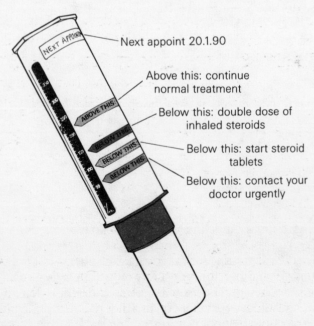

Figure 12.1 Peak flow meter with colour codes

readings will never fall as low as this.

This is all very well in theory, but in practice under extreme stress it can still seem too complicated. I have devised a method of marking the peak flow meters of each asthmatic with a colour system whereby the asthmatic child and the parents will know exactly what steps to take without having to work out percentages. The system takes the form of colour bands which are stuck on to the peak flow meter at the appropriate level for each patient. Simple instructions are written on the band as to what is the correct action. An example of this is shown in Figure 12.1.

After some experimentation we found that the best method was to use colours in the same manner as traffic lights:

- Anything from the green band or better means 'Go'. Everything is alright and maintenance therapy should be continued as normal.
- Yellow for 'Get Ready' and some remedial action should be taken.
- Orange or Amber means that the attack is severe but should still respond to the treatment without the need to call the doctor.
- Red equals 'Stop' and indicates the reading is very low and urgent medical help either from the doctor or at hospital should be sought.

Peak flow meters are vital in the assessment of severity of attacks but it is also imperative to have the right equipment easily to hand at home to deal with any crisis. I have found that all that is needed are the following:

- A bronchodilator inhaler, e.g. Ventolin or Bricanyl.
- A steroid inhaler, e.g. Becotide 50 or Becotide 100.
- A nebulizer, preferably an electric one but a footpump nebulizer will do.
- Bronchodilator nebulizer solution, either Ventolin or Bricanyl.
- A course of cortisone tablets.

If you have all these at home then you will be able to deal with virtually every asthma attack. Since introducing this list plus the colour-coded peak flow meter I have not had to send a child on this régime into hospital. I am sure the reason is that as soon as there is a deterioriation in the peak flow reading suitable action is taken so the level never reaches the red zone.

This list of equipment should be kept in a set place in the home and always kept up to date. The inhalers and nebulizer solution can be readily obtained on prescription from your doctor and you should have no problems maintaining your stock of these. The nebulizer has to be bought and is usually ordered through the surgery. At the time of writing they cost about £85. If this is excessive then a footpump nebulizer is a practical alternative which retails at around £27. The only drawback is the effort required to pump it – and there will be no way your child will be able to do it so it will be down to you!

To my mind every asthmatic child should have access to a nebulizer and certainly from my own point of view it is the best £85 I have ever spent. Not only has it kept my own children out of hospital but it has made them much more self-confident as they know the treatment will work. If you do decide not to buy one then many doctors' surgeries now have them available to borrow. The obvious drawback is that many asthma attacks start at night when the surgery is closed and there is the inevitable delay in starting the treatment until your doctor brings the nebulizer. During this time the wheezing may become much worse. Also it is possible that the machine is already on loan to another patient so there is no possibility of using it, or the attack may start when you are away from home. Some children only experience asthma with a change of environment. It is important when the nebulizer first arrives that you are taught the correct way to use it and I am sure your practice nurse will show you this.

The only slight problem you may experience with this list of equipment is obtaining a course of cortisone tablets. I will discuss how to use them later in this chapter but basically it is a very powerful drug which over a period of time can cause side-effects. However, I have found that to settle an asthma attack it only takes a course of three or four days. Significant side-effects do not occur for about five weeks so there is a wide safety margin. Some doctors argue that they like to see the child before such a strong substance is given, but to my mind this causes delays when further deterioration may occur. Not only that but often if the nebulizer is used as well it may only be necessary to take one or two cortisone tablets. So if your GP is reluctant to give you any, be quietly insistent and I am sure you will be allowed them.

When treating an asthma attack it will obviously depend on how much of this equipment you have at home as to how far down the line you can go. If, for instance, you only have the simple inhalers then you will have to call your doctor as soon as these lose effect, or as soon as the peak flow readings begin to fall through the range of the yellow band.

We can now see how all this information is put into practice with our two children we have followed through this book. Let us take 4 year-old Julie first, as her asthma responds in text-book fashion to the recommended therapy. Her parents had studied my treatment plan following her first serious attack so they were well prepared in the event of a repeat. Julie's precipitating factors were mainly allergies, and following a cold. In this instance it was the aftermath of a cold, so her parents were half-expecting her asthma to start. Her normal peak flow was about 250 and Julie's fell quite quickly to below 200. At that point all they did was to increase her bronchodilator therapy, which she normally took via a Bricanyl inhaler with a spacer tube on the end. In spite of this her deterioration was rapid; within a further two hours her peak flow reading had fallen to 170 and she had become very distressed with shortness of breath and a very troublesome cough.

Julie's mother brought out her electric nebulizer, which she had checked only the previous weekend so she knew everything was ready. A respule of Bricanyl nebulizer solution was twisted open and the contents emptied into the reservoir of the nebulizer. These respules contain a standard dose of the drug. The machine was then switched on and Julie inhaled the cloud of Bricanyl vapour for 10 minutes. Some children prefer a mask but Julie obviously found them too constricting, so used a mouthpiece instead. When breathing in the vapour there is some lost to the atmosphere, but sufficient is always taken into the lungs. At the end of treatment her peak flow had risen back to 210, and although she was still wheezy she looked much better and was not as distressed. Over the following three hours her wheeze again increased and her peak flow fell back to 170, so by the time her next treatment was due Julie was again quite uncomfortable. I often find that it takes more than one dose via the nebulizer to have a lasting effect but the most important point in this case was that the rapid decline in Julie's peak flow readings had been halted.

The dose given through the nebulizer should not be inhaled more than every three hours, otherwise there may be significant absorption into the rest of the body with the risk of unwanted effects. After her next treatment Julie's peak flow reached 220 and only fell back over the next three hours to 195. A further 10 minutes of inhalation brought the level up to 220 again but there was this time no fall-off in her readings. Four hours later her reading was still the same so the parents gave her one more dose and this restored her breathing level to the normal level of 250. The whole attack had needed four doses of the nebulizer and had taken ten hours to settle.

Thus by using the 'big guns' of treatment very quickly, a potentially dangerous situation was averted. If the nebulizer had not been available Julie's parents would have had little choice but to call in their doctor. Also by knowing the treatment had worked Julie developed increased confidence that it would be effective in her next attack.

All through the attack her parents remained calm and unhurried as they followed the treatment plan. They propped Julie upright with pillows behind her back and when she was having the treatment she sat on her mother's knee. Any attempt to lie her down would have made the wheezing much worse. As it was summer it was stuffy in the house so it was advisable to open the window to allow some circulation of air. When she was ill Julie's uncle came to see her. Unfortunately he is a chain smoker; under no circumstances must anyone smoking ciga-rettes be allowed in the same room as a child having an asthma attack. In fact as my own children have asthma neither my wife nor I allow smoking in our house at all. It has only on one occasion caused ill-feeling in one of our friends, but quite honestly if they are prepared to put your child at risk purely to satisfy their own craving then who needs friends like that anyway? Julie's attack responded extremely well to the nebulizer and this was partly due to the speed in which treatment was started. In general terms the length of the attack is directly proportional to the duration of the symptoms. Julie had only been wheezing for just over an hour so she settled very quickly.

Colds certainly were a major factor in Julie's asthma and her next bad episode was at school a few months later. At that time she had been suffering with a sore throat and blocked nose for about four days. One morning at school she started to feel short of breath but did not like to tell the teacher as she would not have been very sympathetic. Consequently her asthma gradually increased through the day until the mistress finally noticed her obvious distress. As it was by this time only 30 minutes before the end of school for the day nothing was done to let the mother know of the situation. When Julie was finally picked up outside the school gates she was in a terrible state and her mother nearly took her straight to the local hospital. However, as she had learnt the treatment plan off by heart she thought she would try one go with the nebulizer first, as Julie would have become hysterical at the idea of staying in hospital.

On arriving home her peak flow reading was down to 105 which was less than 50 per cent of normal, thus classing it as a severe attack. Julie had a constant loud wheeze, her stomach was moving rapidly with her breathing and most worryingly she was becoming very tired. Her attack had been going on untreated for about 5 hours so Julie's mother knew it would take some time to settle. The nebulizer was quickly set up and her mother was thankful that again everything was in place and ready in the kitchen cupboard. Julie herself was relieved to start the treatment but her peak flow afterwards showed only a marginal improvement at 115. At that point her mother phoned me at the surgery and I nipped out quickly between patients to assess the situation.

When I arrived at the house Julie in fact was not showing any of the real danger signs. Her peak flow was only just below 50 per cent mark, she was tired but not totally exhausted and her colour was healthy, with no sign of the worrying blue tinge that can arise on the lips. Just as important was that Julie was quiet and calm, without any sign of restlessness.

I therefore reassured her mother that she had been right to take Julie home rather than to hospital and I was not surprised that the first dose of the nebulizer had only produced a marginal improvement. As I stated above, the longer an attack has been in progress the longer it takes to settle. This wheezing episode had been in progress several hours and there was no way such a serious condition could settle in a few minutes. Julie in actual fact said she felt better and I have noticed this often happens even when the peak flow reading does not alter. The bronchodilator from the nebulizer starts to have some effect only 30 seconds after the start of inhalation and I am sure this is noticed by the child even if it is insufficient to improve the peak flow levels. Her father had now arrived home and I advised both parents to check the peak flow levels every 15 minutes and to let me know if there was any dramatic fall. Really this meant the level falling below 100 which would be nearing the 75 per cent reduction where it can become dangerous. I knew Julie responded well to bronchodilator therapy so was confident I would not hear anything further.

As a precaution I looked in at the house that evening and found that Julie's peak flow had fallen to 100 just before her next treatment was due but a further 10 minutes of inhalation had raised the figure to 125, i.e. to 50 per cent of normal. At the time I was there she was almost ready for her next nebulizer session and a check on her peak flow showed it to have fallen yet again to 100 and her wheezing had again become more pronounced. This time, after another ten minutes inhalation her level again rose to 125. In other words the rapid decline in Julie's condition had been arrested and there were signs of a slight improvement.

I warned her parents that they were in for a broken night as in my experience children will hardly sleep the first night of a severe attack. Usually by the second night there has been sufficient improvement to allow sleep but there will still be some degree of wheezing. This was true in Julie's case as she slept very little that night and by the end of the three hours between treatments had become quite distressed. Gradually, however, her condition improved and her breathing started to quieten down. This was reflected in her peak flow which gradually rose during that first night and through the next day to a level of 190. Julie slept right through the second night and did not require the nebulizer until the morning. Her wheeze had nearly gone and after her breakfast time treatment her flow reading was up to 220. She was then able to use her normal pressurized inhaler until her readings were 100 per cent normal.

Incidentally, as I have already mentioned, if your child ever does fall asleep during an asthma attack don't wake him or her up as the rest will be invaluable and is usually a sign of some improvement. If there is deterioration to anything like a danger level then the child will always wake up.

Julie has subsequently had two or three more quite serious attacks but these have settled extremely well by using her nebulizer and monitoring her peak flow. The one particular lesson to be learnt in her case is that the speed of starting treatment is most important. If she can be 'nebulized' before her peak flow falls below 180 then her recovery is always very rapid. If it falls below this then it takes considerably longer for her breathing to settle down. Her parents have told the school in no uncertain terms the necessity for urgent action and to let them know as soon as any wheezing starts.

Let us now look at Simon's situation; this was more of a challenge as his recovery did not follow a classic course. One of the major reasons for this was that his asthma was precipitated by so many factors and often by more than one at a time. If you can remove the underlying cause of the problem then the attack will settle quicker. A simple example is if wheezing is brought on by exercise, then stopping and resting will help. Similarly, if asthma is caused by an allergic reaction to animals and in Simon's case it was to horses, then moving away from the horses will also make treatment easier. Simon, however, as with so many asthmatics, was allergic to many different factors which made removing the cause extremely difficult.

The other major problem for Simon was that his attacks built up much more slowly than Julie's. He would have a troublesome cough for two or three days followed by a slight wheeze which produced only a small fall in his peak flow. Either Simon wouldn't tell his parents about his slight shortness of breath or else - if he hadn't had an attack for some time - there would be a delay in starting the treatment and a serious attack would develop. As the breathing problem had actually been developing over some time then it would take proportionately longer to settle.

You may remember that earlier in the book I explained that the airways undergo two changes which cause the shortness of breath and wheezing. First, there is the contraction of the muscle in the breathing tubes, known as bronchospasm. Second, the linings of these tubes become swollen and inflamed which produces further narrowing. Julie's attacks were simply the result of bronchospasm, whereas Simon's were a combination of both spasm and swelling. As a general rule bronchospasm comes on quicker but is reversible much faster than swelling.

One particular attack I remember was on a June evening when Simon had been out playing on the school field all afternoon. He had forgotten his morning dose of preventive inhalers and had also had the remains of a summer cold. The combination of this plus the high concentration of grass pollen on the playing field was sufficient to bring on a mild degree of wheezing which did not respond to his pressurized inhalers. Quite suddenly his asthma deteriorated into a severe attack. Once asthma takes a hold then it can develop at an alarming rate and Simon's peak flow fell from 360 to 170 in just thirty minutes.

Obviously this rate of decline caused major worry to his parents. Quickly they assembled the nebulizer but were unable to find the plastic tubing which connected the machine to the reservoir. After a frantic search it was eventually found in their 5 year-old daughter's bedroom where she had been using it as a skipping rope for one of her dolls! This just shows how important it is to take care of this equipment and always make sure when you finish using it that it is cleaned and put away carefully for next time. The treatment of a severe asthma attack is an emergency situation and the last thing you want to be doing is searching for lost pieces of equipment.

Simon took his nebulized Ventolin for the full 10 minutes but did not really feel much better. His peak flow did improve slightly to 190 but this was still less than 50 per cent of normal. It had actually slowed down the rate of deterioration but unfortunately this did not last and within a couple of hours the level was back to 170 and Simon was again very distressed. At this stage his father rang me to see if he could give the Ventolin more often than every three hours. As the nebulizer dose of the drug is about 50 times that of the ordinary aerosol inhaler, giving it too frequently is probably not a good idea. If it was a life-saving measure then it would be worth the chance but Simon's level had not reached the danger level of a 75 per cent drop in peak flow. This would have been around the 100 mark.

When I arrived at the house to see him his peak flow had fallen to 150, although it was almost time for his next nebulizer session. I watched him do this and checked his reading ten minutes later and it showed a rise of only 20 points to 170. In other words although the rate of decline was slowing his asthma attack was becoming slightly worse despite the bronchodilator therapy.

The reason is that Simon was developing swelling of his breathing tubes as well as muscular spasm. Neither Ventolin nor Bricanyl have any real effect on this swelling as they are purely muscle relaxants. The only effective medication to relieve the swelling is the steroid group of drugs, of which cortisone is the commonest. Cortisone has an extremely powerful anti-inflammatory effect which has saved many lives when used in the treatment of asthma. Unfortunately it has been much maligned in non-medical circles because used incorrectly it can lead to troublesome side-effects.

Simon was obviously in need of some steroids to arrest his

asthma attack and I explained this to his parents. There is one major problem with the use of steroids in asthma and that is that it takes three hours to start working and only reaches its peak effect in nine. This means the child does not feel any instant relief.

The only area of controversy is how the cortisone should be given. I normally use a preparation called Becotide, which is available as a nebulizer solution, or Prednisolone which is in tablet form. Some doctors prefer to use nebulizer solution all the time but unfortunately it does not mix with the Ventolin or Bricanyl bronchodilator solutions. Therefore it has to be given following on from the 10 minute bronchodilator inhalation, making 20 minutes of treatment in all and this I find is often too much for the restless child. In fact when I tried it with Simon he was unable to keep the mask on for this length of time.

This is the only instance in the treatment of asthma, other than in young babies, where I recommend the use of medication given by mouth. Cortisone is available in tablet form and its action is very reliable. It need only be used for a short period of time and therefore the possibility of side-effects is very slight. Not only that but as I have already mentioned, by this time the child is in a serious condition and it is imperative that the most effective treatment is given, even at the risk of one or two unwanted reactions.

The cortisone I prescribe is called Prednisolone and is available in tablets of five milligrams. The aim is to start with a high dose to bring the wheezing under control and then to reduce this slowly over a few days to be certain the swelling in the breathing tubes does not recur. In Simon's case he took six 5mg tablets the first day, followed by five the next, four the day after and so on until he finally finished on one tablet a day. Using this method of reducing the tablets by one each day means the course only lasts six days so it is short and over this period is free of side-effects. Indeed a course of these can be repeated several times a year, if necessary, without ill-effects. In a few instances unacceptable wheezing returns within a few days of stopping the Prednisolone. The child, however, will not be too distressed and can then be treated with cortisone in the form of Becotide via the nebulizer.

After Simon had taken his six cortisone tablets we had the difficult task of waiting three hours until they started to take effect. During this time his peak flow fell to 130 but this was corrected to 165 with his next dose of nebulized Ventolin. We were by now well into the night and there was no possibility of Simon falling asleep, so it was a sleepless night for everyone! After another three hours his peak flow had again fallen to 130 but this time reached 190 with the nebulizer. This suggested to me that the cortisone was starting to work and the swelling in the tubes was beginning to diminish. By dawn, when his next treatment session was due, Simon's reading had only dropped to 170 and the nebulized Ventolin raised this to 220. This took him out of the serious band of below 50 per cent and everyone was able to relax. Gradually over the next twenty-four hours, as the cortisone took maximum effect, the readings improved and Simon was able to sleep normally the following night. His treatment sessions were extended to between four and five hours without any fall in readings and generally he felt his breathing was much easier.

Thirty-six hours after the onset of the attack his peak flow was back up to 360 and he was able to continue treatment with his usual pressurized inhalers although he had to complete his course of cortisone. Finally at the end of five days his reading had returned to its normal level of 400.

This usually means that no further acute treatment is needed, although one one occasion when he had finished the Prednisolone his peak flow did fall back to 320, indicating there was still some residual swelling of the airways. We were able to clear this by using Becotide solution in the nebulizer which removed the need to take any further cortisone by mouth.

To summarize: for the treatment of a severe attack in a more resistant case like Simon's, I would first try Ventolin or Bricanyl via a nebulizer. If this does not produce any significant improvement then I would give another dose in three hours. Again if the peak flow readings have only risen slightly I would start a course of Prednisolone tablets in a dose of six per day reducing by one tablet each day. Until the cortisone starts to work I would continue the nebulizer three hourly until the child's condition improves and then start to reduce the frequency of them as long as the peak flow does not deteriorate by doing so. At regular 20-minute intervals when the wheezing is very distressed I regularly check the peak flow to ensure it is not slipping into the danger area. If it falls below 25 per cent of normal then urgent medical help must be sought. The chances of this happening, however, are extremely remote if the steps described above are taken.

This method of treatment shows how important it is to keep a course of cortisone tablets in the house. This can then be given at exactly the right time without having to wait for the doctor to come and then wasting more time going to the chemist to have the prescription made up. Not only that, if the doctor is not experienced in asthma management he may well insist that your child goes into hospital.

As you gain experience with your own child's asthma you will soon realize the most effective treatment that is needed. Julie has needed steroid therapy on only one occasion and usually settles very well on simply using a bronchodilator like Ventolin or Bricanyl in her nebulizer. Simon, on the other hand, nearly always needs cortisone for a bad attack so his parents don't tend to wait until he has used the nebulizer twice. If his peak flow hasn't shown a significant gain after the first treatment then the steroids are started. There is not then a further three hour delay. I must stress, however, that while this is fine for Simon it is not usually necessary, as most children with asthma settle with bronchodilators and never need cortisone.

I am happy to say that although Julie and Simon have had a number of severe attacks they have never needed hospital admission, and their peak flow readings have never reached the danger mark of a 75 per cent fall.

I had stressed to Simon's parents right through his management that it was always my aim to settle his asthma without having to send him to hospital. Simon's father, however, did ask what treatment they give to asthmatics. The peak flow readings are still used as the main guidelines to the severity of the attacks as is the same method of treatment if the asthma is not too severe. The critical time is when there is more than a 75 per cent reduction in peak flow and this is where admission to hospital becomes necessary. In Simon's case where his normal reading was 400 this would mean a reduction to a level below 100.

A fall of this large amount indicates that there is both spasm of the muscles and swelling of the lining of the breathing tubes. The spasm is dealt with in similar fashion to treatment at home by using a nebulizer containing Ventolin or Bricanyl. The swelling is also treated with cortisone but as this takes a minimum of three hours to start working when taken in tablet form, it is given instead by injection. There are basically two ways of injecting medication, either into a muscle or into a vein. In the former it still takes nearly three hours to take effect so the cortisone is always given via a vein in the arm. In this way the drug passes directly into the bloodstream and acts very quickly. It is also possible by this route to administer a much larger initial dose. Injecting into a child's vein is quite tricky and it is impractical to do this at home.

The other benefit of being in hospital is that when the airways are very narrow it is difficult for a child to breathe in sufficient oxygen and the lips will start to turn blue. This will further increase the pressure on the body and rapidly lead to exhaustion. The obvious remedy is to give oxygen through a facemask and then the lips will return to a normal pink colour. The oxygen can be continued until the asthma settles.

Simon's parents did not like the idea of their child being injected and given oxygen but I did stress this would be a life-saving procedure and under those circumstances the treatment didn't seem that bad! Anyway, I let it be a warning to them to make sure they maintained Simon's preventive inhalers regularly and followed the treatment plan precisely when an attack started.

Finally, in this chapter, I would like to mention how the child should be managed when the attack subsides, as both Julie's and Simon's parents asked me about this. If the attack has been mild then normal activities can be resumed straight away. In more severe episodes it is important to take things easy for a couple of days. This not only allows the body to recover its strength but also lessens the risk of another attack developing. Research shows that it does take this amount of time for the blood gases and metabolism to return to normal. The most troublesome symptom in the aftermath is a cough, as there is always an accumulation of thick, sticky sputum. During an actual attack coughing is often suppressed as it may increase breathlessness to an intolerable degree. Unfortunately, as the attack lessens, coughing still seems to exert a narrowing effect on the airways which makes it impossible for the sputum to be brought up.

In the older child like Simon, a simple method of helping is to breathe out against slight resistance; that is, by pursing one's lips as if to whistle and then breathing out in a slow and determined fashion. This technique helps to bring up sputum to the point at which it can be gently coughed up without difficulty. Another way of clearing the mucus is to gently blow one's nose.

I always advise children to avoid violent coughing at this stage as it will increase exhaustion and can actually cause minor damage to lungs that are already very sensitive. In general I have found many of the medicines available which claim to enhance the coughing up of sputum to be of very little value.

Throughout this chapter I have explained the treatment of a severe asthma attack using only the medications that are absolutely necessary. These are summarized in Figure 12.2 and do not actually involve many different drugs, really only a bronchodilator to relieve muscle spasm and a cortisone preparation to settle any swelling of the airway lining. It is the amount and method of administering them that is so important.

I would like to close this chapter by describing the situation of a 6 year-old girl called Kate who was an asthma sufferer. She had just joined my list as her family had recently moved from another part of the country. I asked whether she was on any treatment and this is the list her mother gave me. She was on Ventolin syrup for the muscle spasm, a cough medicine, a sedative medicine to calm her down, an antibiotic to prevent infection, a long-acting bronchodilator tablet, a laxative to counteract the constipation that this tablet was causing, vitamin tablets, a Ventolin inhaler, a Becotide inhaler, an Intal spinhaler and a Bricanyl inhaler in case the Ventolin made her shake. This made eleven preparations in all. I am surprised that Kate could remember which she was supposed to take at what time and I am certain that with this many drugs there was some interaction between them.

I immediately and without hesitation stopped all the medicine by mouth and also her Intal and Bricanyl inhalers. This left her with a Ventolin and Becotide inhaler out of the original eleven. I added a volumatic to make the two inhalers more effective if she became slightly wheezy and her parents agreed to buy Kate a nebulizer. I also prescribed her a course of cortisone tablets to keep at home so they could be used in an emergency. Thus, instead of the original array of medicines and tablets, Kate was managing solely with Ventolin and Becotide which could be given in three different ways depending on the severity of the attack. Hopefully the cortisone tablets would never be needed. Kate had never even heard of a peak flow meter let alone been shown how to use one, so her parents had no way of managing their daughter's condition. Three visits to the asthma clinic at my surgery soon changed that and when I saw Kate a month later

I could immediately sense a much greater self-confidence in her.

I am sure that there are many other children on the same 'hotch potch' of treatment that Kate was on originally, which is far too complicated and totally unnecessary. If your child has asthma it is wise to be under the care of a doctor experienced in the management of this condition. By following this complete treatment plan it is most unlikely you will ever need to summon medical help, but it is always comforting to know it is there if really needed.

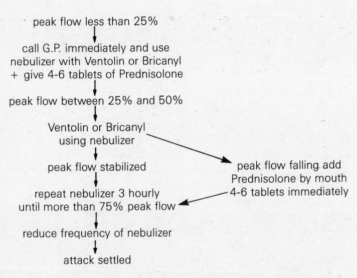

Figure 12.2 Treatment plan for severe attack

CHAPTER 13

Treatment of an Asthma Attack Using Natural Therapy

We live in a changing world and one of the most pleasing aspects is that many people are now trying to treat their ailments by utilizing the body's own healing power, rather than relying on potentially toxic drugs. This is a principle on which I am very keen and would certainly recommend natural therapy whenever possible. The only reluctance I have concerning natural treatment of childhood asthma is that in its severe form it can be life-threatening, so it is vital that the treatment is going to work quickly. Natural therapy does tend to be more gradual in onset and therefore I would not advise using only this when the wheezing is very marked or if the child's condition is deteriorating.

Clare is a 7 year-old who has only ever had mild attacks of asthma but these had recently become much more frequent so that her chest never seemed clear. Her mother was reluctant to put her on regular conventional treatment and asked me which alternative methods I would recommend for the attacks. I have dealt with prevention using natural means in Chapter 8, but Clare really needed something for when she was actually wheezy.

Briefly I reinforced the methods of self-help:

- Turn off the central heating in Clare's bedroom, as it creates currents of air which circulate allergenic particles which Clare would inhale when asleep.
- No smoking by anyone in the house at any time.
- Avoid furry pets and cage birds.
- Take up a sport which will exercise and strengthen the lungs. Swimming is excellent for the development of the rib cage and the secondary muscles of respiration.
- Encourage Clare, who was keen on music, to take up a wind instrument to establish good breathing habits.

I decided to treat Clare with a mixture of acupuncture and homoeopathy as I have found this combination particularly effective in asthma. This means part of the therapy is carried out by a trained specialist as it is obviously an impossibility to carry out acupuncture on yourself; the rest can be your own responsibility by taking the relevant homoeopathic preparation.

Acupuncture

When considering the points to use in acupuncture it is important to consider that actual asthma attacks are associated with deficiencies of energy in the channels of Lungs, Spleen and Kidneys. When a child is wheezing this energy - known as 'Chi' - is prevented from making its normal journey along these channels because of the formation of phlegm and dampness in the lungs. Acupuncture treatment is aimed at relieving wheezing by encouraging the energy to overcome these blockages thus ensuring an unobstructed flow of Chi. I have discussed the theory of acupuncture more fully in Chapter 8.

No child I have ever met likes the thought of needles being stuck in them and Clare was no exception. I reassured her that the needles are very fine and not like those used for injections. Most children have only ever experienced hypodermic needles for their vaccinations and these have to be larger so the immunization fluid can pass down the middle of them. Acupuncture needles do not need this property, so they are incredibly fine, producing virtually no pain when they pass through the skin.

To treat Clare's asthma I used the following points, which I have found to be most effective and which are shown in Figure 13.1. There is one needle inserted at the entry of each channel, the point in the hand being on the top surface between the thumb and first finger and the one on the foot being between the first and second toes. Needling the channels closer to the lungs involves the insertion of a needle at a point quite high on the back and also on the chest below the collar bone and another on the arm below where the triceps muscle covers the shoulder. There is one further point just below the knee which can generally reinforce the flow of energy through the body and it is beneficial to needle this as well. This makes only six points in all, which isn't too many. This is one reason for always seeing

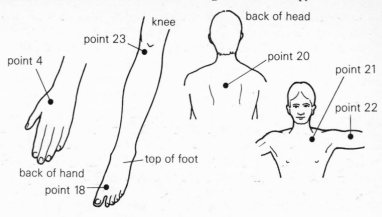

Figure 13.1 6 acupuncture points

an experienced therapist; there are over 50 suggested places to stick in the needles, so an unqualified acupuncturist may use far more points than are really necessary.

Initially, while Clare's asthma was unstable, I treated her once a week. As with conventional medicine I monitored her progress using a peak flow meter. Her usual level was 300 but with this run of wheezing episodes it was hovering around 220. With weekly therapy over five weeks this peak flow rose back to its normal level. I reduced the treatment at that stage to once a month and now some time later all she has is a reinforcing dose every three months.

Acupressure

It is a drawback not being able to do acupuncture at home and for this reason I taught Clare and her mother the technique of acupressure. This works on exactly the same principle as acupuncture, except that the points are massaged instead of needled. This means it will not be as effective as proper acupuncture but it can still be a valuable aid. All that is required is two minutes of firm pressure using either the tip of your fingers or the blunt end of a ball point pen. It is important to remember never to use severe pressure on any of the points - locating the right place is more important than the depth of pressure. As you will be doing it on a child remember you are much stronger than them. Acupuncture points are often very sensitive and it is easy to produce quite marked discomfort.

There are some points described on the abdomen, but I tend to avoid these so there is no risk of damage to the underlying organs. The other important precaution when using acupressure is always to treat children lying down, in case there are reactions such as tiredness or dizziness. Clare didn't really need to use acupressure as her asthma came under control quickly using standard weekly acupuncture. Mark, a 9 year-old who went to the same school as Clare, found that daily acupressure when he was mildly wheezy was the most effective. Massaging the six points I have described for two minutes at a time takes only a total of twelve minutes, hardly an excessive commitment.

Many doctors now practise acupuncture, and I think it is advisable to go to one wherever possible; he or she will be in a better position to advise when it is possible to use acupuncture or when the wheezing is severe enough to warrant conventional medication.

Homoeopathy

This is a form of alternative medicine that I particularly like, as it can be used at home and does not involve any disagreeable procedure on the child. (Not that acupuncture is actually unpleasant but it often produces a degree of fear beforehand.) The one vital factor in asthma is to ensure the correct choice of medication, and so it is not possible, other than by luck, to go and buy a preparation yourself from the local health food shop. Homoeopathy treats the whole person, so it is necessary to consider personality and lifestyle as well as the actual asthma. In my experience it is usual to use one of four possible preparations, depending on the particular symptoms:

- *Arsenicum Album.* When there is great restlessness and exhaustion. The wheezing tends to be worse after midnight and also between one and two in the afternoon. Cold and wet weather is a problem, as is sea air. *Arsen. Alb.* (the abbreviation) is best suited to children who are excessively tidy, intelligent and precise but also have tendencies to fear and anxiety.

- *Ipecacuanha.* The preparation I most frequently prescribe. There is usually a loud rattly cough and associated nausea.

Lying down seems to bring on the breathing problems and the child tends to be a worrier.

- *Kali Bichromicum.* This is used where the symptoms are made worse by noisy surroundings and improve during gentle movement, from warmth, and after nourishment. There is often an associated headache and a loss of voice. The wheezing tends to be worse between three and five in the morning and often leads to nervous exhaustion.

- *Aconite.* Wheezing occurs after exposure to cold, dry wind and is accompanied by great fear. It is also made worse, strangely, by listening to music. Attacks are sudden, violent and brief with a characteristic dry suffocating cough.

Clare was most suited to *Ipecacuanha* and was able to take this on a regular basis instead of her preventive inhalers. The only treatment she is now on therefore is the daily *Ipecacuanha* and occasional acupuncture treatments.

If you do decide to try alternative therapy for asthma it is vital to receive specialist help at the start so the right method is employed. Failure to do this may lead to the wrong choice of preparation which may then not work.

While homoeopathy and acupuncture are my preferred methods of treatment for asthma, there are many other alternative therapies. While it would be perfectly possible to describe them all it would be far too confusing and make it almost impossible to choose the most effective method. There is, however, one story of an 11 year-old called Mandy who is the daughter of a farming couple who always treat their ailments with herbal remedies.

Until the turn of the century the majority of healing throughout the world had a herbal basis and the reason for turning away from herbs was both political and religious. Fortunately some of the great herbalists joined together and published in simple language their knowledge of herbs and healing so that all who read it might seek, find, apply and heal. If a few errors of judgement accumulated here and there it was mainly because of limited knowledge of the condition. Culpeper, in the seventeenth century, produced his *Complete Herbal* which greatly enraged his colleagues at the time as it provided health for the poor; they could go out and search for the relevant herbs freely without having to worry about cost. Herbalism is one form of healing which is virtually impossible to control because anybody nowadays can venture out and collect the plants, make the medicines and take them.

So it was that Mandy was treated with herbs, as her farming family had taken them through several generations. The mixture they gave her was based on the herb Coltsfoot which was originally known as *Tussilago Farfara*. The name *Tussilago* translates into 'cough dispeller' and Coltsfoot has been justly named as 'Nature's best herb for the lungs'. The leaves are actually the basis for British Herb Tobacco although many additional leaves are combined with it including Buckbean, Eyebright, Betony, Rosemary, Thyme, Lavender and Chamomile which are used and smoked for the relief of bronchial troubles like asthma. This tobacco is most beneficial and without the injurious effects as is the case with ordinary tobacco. I mention this purely out of interest and am not suggesting of course that you should give your child something to smoke!

Mandy had her medication prepared as an infusion in the following manner. Her mother mixed together half an ounce each of Coltsfoot, Horehound, Thyme and Grindelia and brewed this with two pints of boiling water, just as you would when brewing tea. To this was added one teaspoon of tinctured or powdered Ginger and thirty drops of Peppermint essence. This was allowed to stand until cool and could then be heated up to drink in acute attacks or taken cold if preferred. To vary the flavour liquorice root or juice, honey or molasses can be added. I am sure that Coltsfoot is the main benefit in this mixture and I know one patient of mine who found she had plenty of Coltsfoot growing near her home so collected it carefully, dried it and then drank an infusion regularly in place of ordinary tea. She continued with this herb alone instead of any other drink and after six months was completely clear of her asthma. Certainly Mandy's condition improved quite dramatically when she took the herb infusion regularly. Her parents had great faith in the herbal mixture and no doubt this belief was passed subconsciously on to Mandy. However it worked it saved her having to take conventional drug therapy. A herbalist friend of mine has also found that Elecampane is effective in asthma in children. This is one of our largest herbaceous plants which is found all over Europe and is widely distributed throughout Britain. It is also called Scabwort or Wild Sunflower. Many years ago it was sold as flat round cakes which consisted of the herb roots, sugar and cochineal colouring. A piece was eaten each night and morning to treat asthma, while it was customary when travelling by a river to suck a piece of root to prevent poisonous exhalations and bad air. The herb is rather bitter for children and is best combined with wild Thyme which makes it far more palatable.

It is exciting that alternative medicine is proving beneficial in treating mild asthma attacks. Certainly the preparation *Ipecacuanha* has proved effective in treating my own son Ross. Always, however, have the stronger conventional medication to hand in case the breathing deteriorates. Hopefully you will never need to use it.

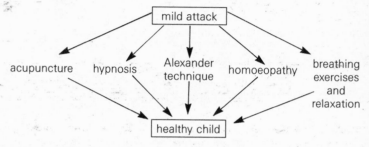

Figure 13.2 Treatment of mild attack using natural methods

Figure 13.2 sums up the various natural methods which can help in the treatment of mild attacks of asthma.

CHAPTER 14

Away From Home

In the previous two chapters I have described the plan for the successful treatment of both mild and severe asthma attacks. This assumes that you are in the comfort of your own house and have all the equipment needed. However, for a good part of the day your child may be away from home, and it is important that any potential breathing problems are anticipated. The three major situations that arise are: at school; when out taking exercise or playing sport; and on holiday. Each of these should not provide any danger as long as certain precautions are taken, so I have dealt with each in considerable detail.

School

The parents of an asthmatic child face two important decisions in relation to schooling. One is whether their child is fit to go to school on that particular day, and the other is what precautions need to be taken actually at school.

The individual decision on whether to go or not will depend to a large extent on the index of severity. A child who has been awake half the night coughing and wheezing is generally in no fit state to go to school the next day. If a cold has led to wheezy bronchitis and the phlegm is turning yellow, it is probably best to allow the child to rest at home. Each mother or father will have their own method of telling; perhaps the speed and ease of washing and dressing, how quickly breakfast is eaten, the sallow tired look, the tinge of blueness in the lips or the pitch of the wheeze. They will know how to balance these criteria against the manipulations of the child. Is homework complete or is there a disliked lesson on that day? Is it games day? If both parents are going out working, then other factors come into play; how will the boss react to another day off? Which parent should stay with the child?

In the end, all these sometimes conflicting forces will result in a decision. Often it will naturally lean towards the side of caution and it will be very irritating on some occasions when the child runs around quite happily all day without much sign of a wheeze. One should remember when this happens that asthma is a potentially life-threatening condition and it is far more important to have a live child than a happy employer! Parents have a built-in protective reflex towards their own children and this should be instinctively followed. If you feel your child isn't fit to attend school then that is usually the right judgement.

Julie and Simon presented different problems when it came to making a decision about school. Julie was in her first term and was much less able to manage her own asthma than an older child. For this reason it was much better in her case to be cautious and keep her off at the slightest sign of a wheeze. In fact her attacks were relatively infrequent and often Julie had recovered sufficiently by lunchtime to go in for the afternoon.

Simon, being older than Julie, was in a different situation altogether. One of the major causes of his attacks was the stress involved in returning to school after the holidays. His parents were therefore reluctant to let him stay off school as it only seemed to prolong the problem. They asked me if there were any definite guidelines I could give them as to whether it was safe to let him go.

Throughout this book I have stressed the importance of the peak flow meter in monitoring the control of asthma in children. Often a fall in readings precedes the start of an attack and using the meter is the only reliable way of telling how breathless the child is becoming. At rest - perhaps sitting at the breakfast table - the breathing may seem quite normal, but as soon as there is any exertion like walking to school the wheezing may be much more apparent. The peak flow meter will give the true picture more clearly. Simon's normal level on the scale was 400. Under no circumstances should he be allowed to go to school if his reading fell below 300, more than a 25 per cent reduction. This reading means moving on to the plan for treatment of an attack as described in Chapters 11 and 12. If his level was somewhere between 300 and 400 then it would be reasonable to let him attend school, as long as his peak flow is stable. In other words it should be measured three or four times between waking up and leaving the house to ensure it isn't falling towards the danger level.

I think it is worth stressing at this point that most children with a mild wheeze actually improve at school. This may be partly because they have been removed from an allergic environment but mainly as a result of the increased discipline in the classroom. The child is kept quietly working at a desk, not allowed to become excited and is also not given too much sympathy. Many is the time I have sent my own son Ross to school with a wheeze and spent the day worrying about him only to see him emerge happy and smiling without the slightest sign of any breathing difficulty.

The exception to this rule is the sensitive child who is frightened of a particular teacher and can start to wheeze in advance of certain lessons. Also, undue pressure from parents to do well academically can induce school-time asthma. As the child strives to reach the standards his mother and father expect during the school day a definite episode of wheeziness can develop and this will only ease as the pressure to perform is lifted. I tactfully suggested to Simon's parents that this could be the case with their son and although they denied it, I am sure it may have been a partial contributory factor.

Equally important as deciding to send your children to school is what action is taken when they are there if a wheezing attack should develop. For a large part of the day they are under someone else's care and it is vital the teachers are able to handle the situation. If you are lucky then the school will have a proper medical set-up. My son Ross is now in his first term at secondary school which has a sick-bay run by a nursing sister. I have donated a nebulizer to the school so I can rest assured that at least he will be well managed should an attack occur at school.

My other children are still at primary school, however and are not so lucky, so what can we do to minimize the risks of problems developing? Parents often complain to me at the asthma clinic that the teachers do not know what to do if a child is wheezy at school. If they are going to be *in loco parentis* for six to seven hours a day then at least they should have some idea how to look after your child. This is a valid point, but rarely in my experience is it really the teachers' fault. Teachers are not doctors or nurses and so do not claim to know a great deal about asthma or any other medical condition. At no stage during their training are they given any teaching on simple medical

conditions and how to react to them. It is up to you as a parent
to protect your child's health at school and to meet the teacher
or nurse and let them know of your child's asthma. They need
to know how often the attacks occur and what brings them on.
Are they affected by exercise and is there anything the child
should not do? The form teacher should have in writing a list of
all the medications that your child takes and how often they
should be given. If you have followed the prevention and
treatment sections in this book then it is unlikely your child is
on more than two inhalers. These seem more acceptable to
teachers than giving medicine. The maintenance therapy is
usually only given twice a day so it may well be that there is no
need for treatment at school on a regular basis.

The most vital information is what action should be taken if
an attack starts. Remember, while these pocket-sized inhalers
will become commonplace to you, most teachers will never even
have heard of them, let alone seen one in action, so please go in
and show the teachers how they are used. The pressurized
bronchodilators like Ventolin and Bricanyl are easy to use and
are most effective in stemming an attack. If you leave precise
instructions as to how many puffs can be given, and if your child
has been properly taught how to use one, then there should be
no cause for alarm.

It is essential both for your child's safety and for the teachers'
peace of mind that they have a telephone number where you can
be reached in an emergency. If you do not do this then you have
to accept that the limited knowledge of the teacher may not be
to the benefit of your child's condition. If you are unavailable for
any reason then it should be made clear that if the school are
worried at all, they should be free to take your child to the nearest
hospital without fear of criticism. Most school teachers are given
little information by parents and are then criticized for not acting
correctly when a problem arises. This is hardly fair on the
teacher. Seeing a child fighting for breath is very frightening so
it is not surprising that teachers tend to panic. I have always
found that if you fully explain a plan of action to them that you
will have very few problems and your child should have a
healthy and happy school life.

Exercise and Sport

Many renowned sportsmen and women have suffered with

asthma in childhood – the cricketer Ian Botham is perhaps the most famous. It should be the aim with all asthmatic children to achieve a degree of control so effective that they are not restricted in any sport they wish to undertake. There are two problems that can arise during exercise, and these are well illustrated by the following two children, both of whom I saw in my asthma clinic recently.

Jayne is a 9 year-old who had suffered with quite severe asthma attacks since the age of 3. She had lived in the middle of Manchester until the age of 8 and I am sure the pollution in the inner city had been mainly responsible for her frequent wheezing episodes. Since moving to a more rural area her asthma had considerably improved and because of this Jayne became rather lax at using her inhalers. Although she no longer had any major attacks Jayne often found that she was short of breath and wheezy when doing games at school. Netball was not too bad but worst of all was cross-country running, which basically consisted of two laps around the school field. The first lap was usually alright but she became very short of breath on the second and usually had to stop and walk.

On checking her peak flow at rest I discovered that it was 325 when her predicted level was 375. During exercise more oxygen is needed by the muscles and therefore the lungs have to work harder. If the breathing tubes are already narrower than they should be, then the lungs have to work even harder to take in the extra oxygen, so the shortness of breath becomes more severe and the wheeze more pronounced. Jayne therefore was an example of a child whose asthma in general was poorly managed and this showed itself when she exercised. All that was needed in her case was to make sure that her preventive inhaler – Becotide 50 – was taken in the correct dose of two puffs twice a day. In fact I noticed from her case records that she had not had a new inhaler for nearly three months, indicating that Jayne had hardly been using it at all. An average inhaler contains 200 puffs and at 4 puffs a day should last 50 days, less than two months. When she went back to the recommended dosage her peak flow rose to 395 which then left her plenty in reserve for when she exercised. She is now able to complete two laps of the school field without any sign of problems.

There is also a specific condition called 'exercise-induced asthma'. Certain asthmatic children, although able to exercise perfectly freely, find they become increasingly wheezy when the exercise has finished. Twelve year-old Neil was typical in that he was very keen on all sport but – particularly after a hard cross-country race at school – he found that his asthma was very troublesome. Everyone becomes short of breath on exertion but this normally settles quickly when the exercise is finished. However Neil found that, instead of being able to relax and 'get his breath back', a paroxysm of wheezing would overtake him. This is proof of exercise-induced asthma, as no other form of chest disease is associated with breathlessness which becomes worse immediately after the exercise has finished. With Neil the wheezing reached a peak after a few minutes and could take up to an hour before there was any relief, even when using his inhalers.

During the course of exercise it is difficult to make accurate measurements of the width of the airways. However, the information that is available does suggest that in most people, including asthmatics, the airways actually widen during exercise, i.e. the peak flow increases. It is what happens after that provides the crucial difference. In normal people, the airways quickly revert back to their previous state, but in the asthmatic this is not so. For some reason the airways continue to narrow for up to five minutes, remain at that level for some time and then slowly widen out again. The extent of the change can be quite considerable and certainly this was the case with Neil. His normal resting peak flow reading was 450 but when measured five minutes after the end of a gruelling cross-country race at school it had fallen to 220. In other words there was a 50 per cent reduction in lung capacity in just five minutes, so it was not surprising that Neil was so distressed.

Exercise can be taken in many different ways and not all appear to be equally potent stimuli for exercise-induced asthma. In some children simply jumping about in the bedroom is sufficient stimulus and I have known my own son Ross to wheeze after the effort of laughing at a comedy programme on television. Both Jayne and Neil developed it after running and certainly I have found this to be the commonest precipitating cause. Indeed, only six to eight minutes of running is needed to bring on a severe attack of asthma and many will become wheezy in less time than this. Cycling will also produce breathing problems but less consistently, perhaps because only the legs are used. Swimming seems to be the most innocuous of all and can be recommended to everyone with asthma. In everyday life the asthmatic child will find that the severity of wheezing is less with shorter periods of exercise and with light as compared to heavy exertion. Quite hard sports, for example playing football or cricket, can be tolerated by the asthmatic, provided it is in brief bursts with some respite in between.

Almost all asthmatic children have exercise-induced asthma, so what can be done to prevent it? Without becoming too technical, it seems that an attack comes when the muscles of the airways are stimulated by the release of chemical substances. Exercise causes the release of these chemicals, but they have not yet been identified. It is interesting to note that if further exercise is taken within one or two hours then the degree of wheezing produced is much less. This suggests that the first bout of exercise depletes the stores of these chemicals and that it takes some time for them to be replenished.

The prevention of exercise-induced asthma is very simple: as it is caused by muscle spasm a dose of one of the bronchodilator drugs is the treatment of choice. You will remember that this can be given either in the form of Ventolin or Bricanyl through a pressurized inhaler, a turbohaler, a rotahaler or a diskhaler. While it can be given when the child becomes wheezy it is far more effective if given just prior to the exercise starting. Let us consider this in practice with the case of 12 year-old Neil above.

Neil's main preventive medication was a Becotide inhaler. It has no real effect on muscle spasm, so increasing the dose would not prevent exercise-induced asthma. His main bronchodilator or anti-spasmodic was Bricanyl and by taking three puffs of this just prior to running Neil found that he was virtually free of wheezing after the race. Unfortunately he found that the Bricanyl, as it does in some children, made his legs feel weak and tired. While this was of no consequence in normal living it reduced his running performance. By switching to a Ventolin inhaler Neil found his running times improved. Ventolin has the side-effect of producing a slight tremor; this is harmless but in school Neil found it affected his writing. It did not, however, make any difference to his running. He was in a situation therefore of using a Bricanyl inhaler for normal wheezing episodes and a Ventolin inhaler for his exercise-induced asthma. Occasionally if it was before an important race he would use Ventolin via a nebulizer before leaving home. Personally I doubt if this is really necessary as the simple inhalers are most effective and I suspect with Neil there was an element of nervous asthma related to the tension of a big event.

In summary, the key to preventing exercise-induced asthma is to give a bronchodilator about ten minutes before exercise begins. This sounds easy but in younger children is often forgotten, especially at school. It is important to discuss this carefully with your child's teacher so your son or daughter does not feel self-conscious or embarrassed about using it. Whichever bronchodilator your child normally uses should be used to prevent the exercise-induced asthma, i.e. it can be a pressurized inhaler, a turbohaler, a rotahaler or a diskhaler. Always remember that exercise is not harmful to an asthmatic child. It is very often frustrating and annoying not to be able to engage in vigorous sports because of shortness of breath. Physical fitness is as beneficial – if not more so – to an asthmatic child as it is to anyone else. For this reason this important aspect of asthma control should never be ignored.

Holidays and Staying Away from Home

In my surgery and in the asthma clinic one of the factors that causes great concern to parents is whether it is safe to go on holiday. My answer is invariably 'yes', as it is important for a child with asthma to lead as normal a life as possible. I have a young teenage patient who is going to Kenya on her third safari this year! The only time I would recommend staying at home is if the asthma is in an unstable condition. If attacks are coming very frequently it is wise to have the treatment reviewed and appropriate action taken in the stable environment of your own home. Usually this does not take long and hopefully only means a postponement of the holiday rather than a total cancellation. For the vast majority of asthmatics it is perfectly safe to go away but as a precaution you must ensure that you have the means to deal with an attack if one should occur.

Most vital is to remember to take the medication with you! This may sound silly but for three years I worked in a hospital in Blackpool and we once calculated that over half our admissions in summer were people who had forgotten to bring their medicine with them. Inhalers are usually the last to be packed so they can be easily reached and it is amazing how often they are left behind on the bedroom table. Also make sure you have one or two spare inhalers with you as they do have an irritating habit of running out or being lost just when needed most. If you are staying in this country then an attack can almost be as easy to treat as at home. It is well worth remembering to check when you arrive at your destination as to where the local doctor is based and how to make contact in an emergency. Everyone in the United Kingdom is entitled to medical treatment wherever they are staying free on the N.H.S. If you are staying in a hotel – and this applies particularly in London – the staff will often call a doctor privately for you, and the visit plus treatment can take up most of your holiday spending money. You are within your rights to ask for an N.H.S. visit and you should always insist on this. A useful tip is to take your own doctor's phone number away with you and give him or her a ring first for advice. It is not very often necessary to call a doctor out, especially if you follow the treatment plan laid out in this book.

The first night of a holiday is the one when your child is most likely to suffer an asthma attack as the change of environment throws up different kinds of allergens and also there is all the excitement. So be organized and unpack the medication before you retire to bed.

If you are travelling abroad the situation is slightly more complicated, though if you are well prepared you should have little trouble. First, before you go, make sure you have adequate medical insurance just in case you need it. If you are going to the United States also ensure you have a credit card with sufficient reserve funds on it, as often the hospitals over there want the money before they will give the treatment. The last thing you want at that time is to have the stress of ringing insurance companies to obtain a cash advance.

One of my patients, a little 5 year-old called Victoria, recently had to be admitted to a hospital in Italy with an asthma attack because her parents had not taken her nebulizer with them. I agree it is very bulky and difficult to fit into a suitcase but it does have a carrying handle. To me it is the most vital piece of luggage and must have top priority. Most people take far too many clothes away with them, so leave some behind and take the nebulizer instead.

Taking a nebulizer away with my own children has completely transformed our holidays, as it has taken all the anxiety away over the possibility of being unable to treat an attack. If it is combined with the use of a peak flow meter then it will be rarely necessary to use any local medical facilities. If there is any doubt before you leave about the power supply then it is wise to take a foot pump nebulizer rather than an electric one. These are cheap to buy or often your own doctor will lend you one to take with you. It is no use if your child has an asthma attack and there is nowhere to plug in the nebulizer!

Just one word of warning: always tell the customs office what the machine you are carrying is used for. Eleven year-old James arrived back at Gatwick from Florida with his father carrying the nebulizer. The customs officer must have thought he was a drug smuggler, because he completely stripped the machine down, causing all kinds of damage and rendering it completely unusable.

Equally important to take with you is a course of cortisone tablets, and I would recommend taking them very early in an attack. When you are away from home it is often difficult to tell how severe an attack is going to be and anyway you want to enjoy the holiday. The sooner the attack settles the better for everyone, so it is worth starting the cortisone as soon as the wheezing starts. Using 5mg tablets, a loading dose of two tablets followed by one tablet three times daily is quite adequate. Your own doctor will, I am certain, supply you with these before you go.

Should you by any chance forget to take any of the medication, then do not despair. Most foreign countries have a much more relaxed approach to selling medicines than here and most are available over the counter. I remember going to Skiathos, a small Greek island, having forgotten to take any cortisone tablets with me. It was before the island had been developed for tourists so I was a little concerned when I sought out the local pharmacy. There was no cause for concern because their stock was larger than most chemists over here and there were several types of cortisone to choose from!

So, when you go on holiday try and keep calm and resist the urge to panic. This is not easy when you are in a foreign land and so many miles from home. If you go well prepared then management should be straightforward. Remember also that it is easy to ring home these days so take your doctor's phone number with you. Last summer I had calls from Hong Kong and Brazil - unfortunately no one has so far offered to fly me out to treat them!

As a final note on holidays, I am often asked about air travel.

This will only cause problems in those with such severe and disabling asthma that oxygen levels in the blood are already low. A reduction in oxygen in the air in the aircraft cabin occurs at high altitude and at six thousand feet can be as much as 25 per cent. This could cause some embarrassment to the severe asthmatic and increase breathing difficulties. Fortunately oxygen is readily available. I must stress, however, that this will very rarely be needed and I would have no qualms about taking a child with asthma in an aeroplane.

The other difficult situation to face is when your child is asked to stay at a friend's house or with a relative. Sleeping in another bedroom can carry risks as the amount of dust may be different and the pillows may be feather, both of which increase the allergic response and may produce wheezing. Other questions are: do they have any pets? Will your child become over-excited? Will he or she be too frightened to wake anyone if wheezing develops at night? In reality, if your child's asthma is well controlled it is most unlikely that any problems will arise. I remember 4 year-old Julie's parents spending a virtually sleepless night the first time she stayed at a friend's house. Julie was perfectly alright with not the slightest hint of a wheeze. It is most important to ensure that all the normal medication is sent with the child and whoever is going to be the guardian knows exactly what action to take if wheezing should develop. I have found there is little point in simply telling friends or relatives, as under pressure they often can't remember what to do. Far better is to write it all down step by step so they have an easy procedure to follow. Furthermore, if you are really worried then make sure you can be contacted if necessary. Simon's parents were worried because he was booked into an activity camp for a week's holiday in the summer and they were concerned that he would be out of contact for so long. Once again I advised them to make sure Simon had his inhalers and nebulizer with him and to explain to the nurse at the camp about the potential problem. Simon did have a minor attack half-way through the week but this was easily treated with extra doses of Ventolin and he had a tremendous holiday.

It is always worrying leaving your own child in someone else's care, but it is vital that an asthmatic child is allowed to lead a normal life. If you prevent them from going then this will cause resentment which may lead to far more stress and tension in the end.

CHAPTER 15

Your Questions Answered

When the doctor tells you that your child has asthma it does come as quite a shock. Many questions crowd the mind at the same time and there is little or no time to ask them. More thoughts will occur to you on the way home or over the subsequent weeks and it isn't easy to have them answered in the rush of a busy surgery. Even when you have become an 'expert' in treating your child's attacks there will still be situations when you are not sure of the correct action to take. In this chapter I have provided answers to the questions that I am most frequently asked in the surgery or at home. There may occasionally be some overlap in areas I have covered earlier in the book but it may be difficult at a glance to find the exact answer in the main body of text. I have deliberately kept the replies as brief as possible so they can be used for quick reference.

Is asthma inherited?

Undoubtedly there is often a history of allergy either in the form of hay fever or asthma in one or both parents. So the tendency to develop the condition is at least partly inherited, and is then actually brought on by either infection, pollution, further allergy or stress.

Can babies develop asthma?

Asthma can develop in babies although it is uncommon below the age of twelve months. Many babies develop a sort of wheezy bronchitis which is not true asthma and which is often a 'one-off' event. Croup, which is a throat infection, can mimic asthma but responds to steam inhalation. It is the recurrent nature of the wheeze which tends to confirm asthma in babies, as many will have only a single episode and never wheeze again.

Will my child grow out of her asthma?

It is the increased irritability of the airways that is the root problem in asthma and fortunately this does settle down gradually as the child's age increases. Many have grown out of the condition by the age of 12 although for some it can take longer. The factor that is most vital is to keep your child free of attacks for as long as possible, to allow the airways to become less sensitive. If there is frequent wheezing, perhaps once or twice a month, then there is little chance of the condition settling spontaneously. This is one of the reasons why it is so important to take preventive medication on a regular basis.

How do I explain to my daughter that she has asthma?

Firstly, always use the word asthma to describe what is wrong with her. It does not help to use vague expressions. Many children, even when very young, will know another child with asthma but will only relate to them if they know that they have it as well.

Explain to your daughter how the air passes from the nose and mouth into the lungs, perhaps likening them to balloons which go up and down as the air goes in and out. I always liken the airways to drinking straws through which the air travels to the lungs. In asthma the problem is that these tubes become narrowed rather like a straw that has been bitten and chewed. This makes it more difficult to drink through and less liquid comes up the straw. In the same way, less air flows out of the lungs or balloons because the airways or straws are narrowed. Medicines need to be taken to make these straws become wider and the most effective way is to use an inhaler or 'puffer' which sprays a fine jet of medicine straight on to the straws themselves. Occasionally if the asthma is bad enough this spray has to be breathed in through a mask for ten minutes.

My child has to use inhalers twice a day, every day. Is it safe to do this?

Most definitely. The reason is that the dosage used in medication that is taken straight into the lungs is ten times less than in drugs that are swallowed. Inhaled drugs go straight to the breathing tubes which are the problem area, whereas swallowed drugs have to circulate all round the body, including places like the heart, brain, liver and kidneys. These can produce side-effects in any of these parts, whereas by using inhalers there is negligible absorption into the rest of the body and so side-effects, if they occur at all, are only very slight. This is the reason why I have emphasized the importance right through this book of using inhaled medication rather than tablets or medicine.

What about cortisone?

This to some people is a dreaded word, as when the drug was first produced it was thought to be a complete cure for virtually everything and consequently was often prescribed irresponsibly for too long a period. Side-effects developed and left everyone very suspicious of it. I must stress, however, that used correctly for short, sharp courses it is a most valuable and effective drug. Its main action is to reduce the swelling of the lining of the airways, and this can be a life-saver. Furthermore if used pro-phylactically, via an inhaler, cortisone can prevent asthma attacks developing. The absorption into the rest of the body is negligible, so no unwanted effects can develop. In severe attacks cortisone is given either as a single injection or in tablet form for a few days. Research has shown that it takes at least five weeks of continuous treatment to produce any significant ill-effects. So please do not worry if your child is put on to treatment containing cortisone.

Are the medications addictive?

They most certainly are not, and if your child seems to require more and more of the inhalers then a review of the treatment is needed. It usually means there is either poor inhaler technique or the dose needs raising as the child grows older.

Will my child become immune to the medication?

There is no loss of effect with continuous usage, so again if your child seems to need larger doses then the treatment needs reviewing, especially inhaler technique.

My child always has a nasty cough during an attack. Would you recommend using a cough medicine?

As the airways are very irritable it does make the child cough continuously. Coughing is a very strong reflex action whose main purpose is to protect the lungs from dust and grit. To completely dampen this reflex would leave the lungs wide open to any foreign particles which are breathed in. Unfortunately most cough medicines are only soothants which do not affect this reflex and therefore have little effect. The real key in controlling the cough is to settle the wheezing.

What is the maximum number of medications my child should take?

A newly-registered patient of mine came for review of her treatment at our asthma clinic and I found she was on eleven different types of medicines, tablets and inhalers. In my experience it is always possible to control asthma using a bronchodilator inhaler, a cortisone inhaler, a nebulizer and a course of cortisone tablets. Therefore the maximum number of different drugs, even in a severe attack, is four and for routine use or in milder episodes should only be one or two.

Is it safe to exceed the stated dose?

With drugs taken via an inhaler there is a wide safety margin so in general it is not dangerous to take extra. As I mentioned above the dose of the inhaler is only one tenth that of a corresponding tablet and in fact is only one fiftieth of that produced via the nebulizer. It is not the worry of toxic effects in increasing the dose that is important but rather the indication that a change in treatment is needed.

How can you tell if the inhalers are nearly empty?

If you are using a diskhaler or rotahaler then it is easy to see how many disks or capsules are left. The sealed pressurized inhalers are more difficult as the drug is in a vapour form. My son devised a trick to give some indication. By placing the cannister of the inhaler into a bowl of water the position of it shows how much remains. If the cannister sinks then it is nearly full, if it points directly down it is half full and if it floats flat then the cannister is empty. Of course it is always wise to have a spare inhaler readily available in case of emergency. Not only do they become empty just at the vital moment but they also have the irritating habit of suddenly refusing to work, even if they are nearly full.

When should I call the doctor?

Basically you should seek help any time you are worried that the treatment is not working. Hopefully if you follow the plan laid out in this book you will never have to call your GP, but never be afraid to do so. If it is during the daytime then wherever possible you should take your child to the surgery as all the equipment and facilities will be readily available there. If it is out of hours then ask for a home visit. Most doctors, if you are pleasant, will willingly come and see your child, but try to be reasonable with your request. Only last week I was called out at two in the morning to a child with asthma who had been wheezing since early evening. His parents had delayed the visit request until they had been to a party!

The other positive reason to seek help is if the peak flow readings are falling rapidly, and particularly if it reaches a level which is less than 25 per cent of normal. This usually coincides with your child developing a blue tinge to the lips and becoming exhausted. It is better to play safe than to regret it afterwards.

What if the doctor refuses to visit?

Many people do not realize that they do not have a right to a home visit and it is the doctor's decision whether to visit or not. Of course, if a visit request is refused and something happens to your child then you can sue the doctor for negligence, but that won't bring your child back. Therefore, if your GP does decline to come out I would have no hesitation in bundling your child into the car and going to the nearest casualty department. If you haven't your own transport then dial 999 for an ambulance. By doing this you risk your child being admitted to hospital but this would probably only be overnight and again it is better to be safe than sorry. I must stress, however, that the vast majority of doctors will gladly visit a child with an asthma attack.

Should we see a specialist?

This is a difficult question to answer, as really if your child's asthma is well controlled and not interfering with his or her life then there is no real indication to see a specialist. Some parents like the reassurance a consultant will give so if you feel you would like this yourselves then by all means ask to see one. Much will depend on how much confidence you have in your own doctor. If the asthma attacks are frequent and your GP does not take any corrective action then a visit to a specialist would seem advisable.

Are desensitizing injections worth having?

The general answer to this question is no. There are two main reasons: first, they usually consist of eighteen weekly injections which can be painful, no child that I have ever met likes needles and it is unfair to subject anyone to this number; second they often are not effective. Asthma is rarely precipitated by a single allergy, so being desensitized to only one allergen will not prevent attacks occurring. The only possible justification is if your child is particularly sensitive to one animal (perhaps the family dog) and it would cause more heartbreak to give it away than to have the injections.

Can we keep pets?

Pets are one cause of asthma and may be blamed unnecessarily. If you have a child with asthma then I would not buy any new animals. This may sound harsh but it is important to remember that asthma can be a life-threatening condition and it would be reprehensible to place your own child's life at risk purely for the sake of keeping a cat or dog. If you already have a pet and the asthma attacks are uncontrolled then the only action to take is to give it a holiday with a friend or in kennels. If the asthma decreases greatly then it may be necessary to part with the pet. If there is no change then obviously the asthma is not pre-cipitated by animal dander.

Should my child eat a special diet?

Certainly by boosting the immune system your child will be better able to fight off an impending attack. This means eating a fresh wholefood diet free of additives and taking a daily multivitamin supplement. In asthma there is always the possibility of a food allergy, although in my experience this is usually fairly obvious because the symptoms occur soon after eating or drinking the offending substance. Thus if your child has a wheezing episode try to work out what has been recently ingested. Preservatives in food can also cause problems, the commonest of which are tartrazine and monosodium glutamate. These should be avoided wherever possible.

Should we move house to a cleaner area?

There is no indication that moving to a different area makes the slightest difference in the incidence of asthma, unless of course you move to the top of Mont Blanc where there is no dust. Those who do emigrate or try a different area are usually bitterly disappointed at the results and much worse-off financially. Not only that but there is the inevitable psychological effect on the child at moving to a new school and having to make new friends.

Does my child need a special school?

No. There is absolutely no indication for this and it is vital that any child with asthma should be treated as any other child would be.

Are there any sports that will help asthma?

Swimming is an ideal sport and should be encouraged in every child with asthma. Adrian Moorhouse, the Olympic and Commonwealth gold medallist, had quite severe asthma when a youngster and firmly believes taking up swimming was mainly responsible for the improvement in his condition. Furthermore the warm humid air of swimming baths does not irritate asthmatics and the exercise of swimming, with its breathing control, is of great benefit.

What activities should be avoided?

The answer is probably none, but really it is a matter of common sense. In some children a certain exercise may bring on wheezing. I know one child who was perfectly well controlled except when he went to karate lessons. Since he was quite happy to stop going to these there seemed little point in increasing his preventive medication just for this purpose. If your child is particularly keen to do a certain exercise then it should be possible to control the wheezing but there is no real point in striving for this only to find he or she is not too concerned about giving it up. In my experience cross-country running is the sport most likely to induce an attack and this should not be forced on asthmatic children against their will.

What precautions should be taken when choosing a career?

For the majority of asthmatic children there should be little restriction when planning a future career. There are, however, three important precautions to consider. First, if specific allergies are known to exist, an occupation exposing the asthmatic to these allergens is obviously to be avoided. Those sensitive to pollen shouldn't become landscape gardeners and there is little point in working in a zoo if attacks are brought on by animals. Second, if asthma is induced by exercise it may be wise to avoid occupations that are particularly strenuous. This is not imperative, however, as it should be possible to control any asthma triggered by exertion. Third, any job where there is smoke, air pollution, irritating fumes or dust should be avoided if possible. This includes such trades as baking and carpentry and working in public houses with their inevitable smoky atmospheres. I have not in any way meant this list to sound restrictive as I am a firm believer that everyone should follow the career they will enjoy the most, and this applies just as much to asthmatics as to anyone else.

Is it safe to wear woollen clothing?

Few special rules need to be made about clothing, unless there is also eczema when irritating fabrics, especially wool, will need to be avoided. Dust fragments trapped in fluffy clothing can irritate the asthmatic child's airways and chemical detergents used in washing may trigger allergies. The particular allergy which arises from biological washing powders, however, has not been shown to produce a sufficiently strong enough allergic reaction to cause a wheezing attack. Keeping reasonably warm in cold weather is sensible, but there is no evidence that concentrating the warmth about the chest by wearing a thick vest makes the slightest difference in asthma.

Apart from giving all the prescribed medication, what should I do when my child has an attack?

There is nothing more frightening to a child than being unable to breathe so the first rule is to appear calm yourself. Ensure that whatever inhalers you have been advised to give in an attack are administered correctly and at the right time. If the child is too distressed to synchronize the firing of the inhaler then do it for them. Watch the breathing in and out and press the inhaler just as the breath in starts and tell the child to hold their breath for a minute. There is a certain magic to children in inhaling medication and if you reinforce this with reassuring words then the effect will be doubled. Make sure the nebulizer is set up ready for the next treatment so there is no extra distress caused by searching for the bits to it.

Make the child comfortable, sitting upright either in a chair or on the edge of the bed. Encourage him or her to relax and breathe slowly. Remind him or her of breathing exercises they have been taught and make sure they are used. Something to occupy the child's mind is useful, this might be television, a record, a story or a puzzle. All the time emphasis should be on an outward quiet confidence and an inward alertness.

Should we avoid emotional upsets in our child?

When your child is correctly treated there should be complete control of his or her asthma. With this control any child can throw a tantrum, rant and rave or laugh heartily without any deterioration in the chest condition. If there is not total control then such events may well bring on a bout of wheezing. Rather than wrap your child up in cotton wool it is better to go for optimum control of symptoms. So do not become over-protective as this will not help your child's emotional development. Having decided on this principle it is still worth not inviting trouble by trying to anticipate any problems that may develop. Simon, the boy we have followed through this book, often became emotionally upset in the couple of days before returning to school after the holidays. His parents, by giving him massive reassurance during this period were able to stop any attacks developing at this time. If your own child does have a degree of emotional asthma try to identify the causes for this and discuss them.

At what time of day is it best to use the inhalers?

This obviously depends on the severity of the asthma. If it is mild then it is usually controllable by giving medication in the morning and evening. This makes the whole condition much simpler to manage as it is reasonably easy to remember treatment when you get up and when you go to bed but surprisingly difficult in the day. If the asthma is more severe then it may be necessary to take the medication to school. A metered aerosol is small enough to be carried in a pocket and can be used when necessary.

Will the school usually be able to give the medication?

I have dealt with schooling at some length in Chapter 14, but briefly the answer to this question is 'yes', as long as the teacher has been told exactly what to do and has it clearly written down as to the exact medications that your child is taking and how often they should be given. Also remember that asthma can be very frightening to teachers and most of them are given far too little information by parents and are then criticized for not acting correctly when a problem arises.

My husband smokes cigarettes at home. Will this affect my child's asthma?

For the asthmatic there is only one rule about smoking: Don't! Irritability of the airways is a fundamental fault in asthma. To irritate them further with cigarette smoke is stupid. Tests have clearly shown that living in a house with a smoker is almost as bad for the child as actually smoking a cigarette themselves. This is a perfect opportunity for your husband to give up himself and make the house a generally much purer place to live. It amazes me how often I am asked this question and how disappointed most smokers are with the answer!

We are bringing our children up the French way and allowing them a little wine with their Sunday lunch. Will it do them any harm?

It is surprising how often I am asked this question and I must admit my own children have had a tipple occasionally since very young. Alcoholic beverages feature all too frequently in the list of triggers for asthma. The alcohol itself is not the culprit but rather the additional components that give a drink its distinctive flavour. Whether the mechanism is allergic or chemical is not known but whatever the reason, sensitivity to alcoholic drinks can be one of the most annoying features of asthma in later life. As white wine has the least additives I would stick to this for your children and not be tempted to give stronger spirits!

My daughter's asthma has suddenly become more troublesome after several years of good control. She has been to the asthma clinic but adjusting her medication hasn't helped. Can you suggest anything?

If the inhalers do not bring the expected control it is important to work through the following checklist:

- Remember to check that all treatment routines are correctly followed.
- Make sure your child's inhaler technique is correct. Often children do it in a rush and do not allow sufficient time for the drug to be absorbed before breathing out. This is the commonest cause of failed treatment and if in any doubt do call in to your surgery and ask the practice nurse to check the technique.
- Keep all dust, smoke and animal danders to a minimum.
- Stop all cigarette smoking in the house and ask friends at their houses not to smoke when your child is there.
- Do discuss and air fully any worries and fears your child may have. It is surprising how often emotions can upset the balance in asthma.
- Boost your child's immune system by ensuring she eats a fresh wholefood diet, takes regular exercise and has sufficient sleep and relaxation. Building up the natural body defences is vital in the effective control of asthma.

- Make sure your child isn't eating too many foods with preservatives, flavourings and colourants in as these can trigger asthma attacks.

I am so fed up with my son taking all these drugs. Can I change him to alternative medicine?

More and more people are becoming bothered about taking modern drugs as all of them seem to have side-effects of one sort or another. I am one of the greatest supporters of alternative medicine and wherever possible in my practice I will treat both children and adults by natural means. For this reason I detailed the different therapies available for preventing asthma in Chapter 8. It is also quite feasible to use natural methods for treating a mild attack and I have described them in Chapter 13. However, I would not risk using them in a severe episode, either where the peak flow is less than 50 per cent of normal or where the child's condition is deteriorating rapidly. This is really because their effect tends to be more gradual and time is of an essence where the breathing is very distressed. So by all means try alternative methods for prevention and for non-serious situations but do not hesitate to change back to conventional methods if the asthma becomes severe.

My doctor has just started an asthma clinic. Is this worth going to?

I must say that since I started an asthma clinic at my own surgery the control in all the children who attend has greatly improved and in fact none of them has had to go into hospital. The benefits are mainly simple ones in that the main problems in asthma arise from children either not taking their medication regularly or from using the inhalers incorrectly. By coming to a clinic and having their peak flow regularly recorded it is easy to see when things are starting to go wrong and often this is before the child or parents are aware of any change, so action can be taken before the child shows any sign of a wheeze. Inhaler technique can be checked and any adjustments made to this when necessary. It may be as your child reaches a different phase of development that a new type of inhaler is required. Also with advancing technology your child can be switched to a more up to date therapy very quickly.

Perhaps the greatest benefit is the reassurance that these clinics give to both child and parents. For a clinic to be effective it must be an open-access type where no appointment is needed. My own asthma clinic consists of myself and two practice nurses. These nurses have been on courses specifically training them in asthma and its management and are now very experienced in the problems that arise in management. Thus if parents feel worried they can call in at any time and see either the nurses or myself to discuss the appropriate action. Being secure in the knowledge that they have professional back-up at all times actually gives them far more confidence. So I would certainly recommend giving it a try.

Are there any asthma associations we can join?

In many chronic diseases, parents have found considerable mutual benefit in meeting together and discussing difficulties and sharing successes. Local doctors, nurses, social workers, natural therapists and others often attend these meetings to explain aspects of the disease, answer questions and generally stimulate interest. Fund-raising is nearly always a feature of these groups and the money is channelled to some central advisory body to be allocated for educational or research purposes. The Asthma Research Council was formed over fifty years ago and has concentrated its activities in raising funds for research in the hope that a cure can be found. There are many other groups that exist in all parts of the country that are more concerned with friendship and support rather than fund-raising. I am sure there will be one in your area and either your own doctor or the local library should be able to give you a contact number. Local groups are not to the liking of everyone but they can be most helpful and certainly provide a way of discussing problems.

CHAPTER 16

The Future

Asthma is now thought to affect 10 per cent of children in this country and no doubt similar numbers throughout the world. However, it is very important for children and parents to realize that for the vast majority it is a mild, albeit annoying illness. It should be seen more as an inconvenience than as a disease which is going to interfere with the child's lifestyle and development.

Wherever you go there are success stories to show asthma can be beaten and allow a normal lifestyle. Many famous athletes, including cricketer Ian Botham and Olympic gold medallist Adrian Moorhouse have never let it affect their sport. There are internationally famous rowers, footballers, dancers, opera singers and actors with asthma who have refused to let their wheezing affect their performance.

As well as the famous there are very many boys and girls who have suffered serious breathing difficulties but for whom asthma is no longer a problem. Many of these children run and play at games without the slightest sign of asthma but occasionally need a little help from their medication. As they know that their inhalers are effective they need only pause for a few seconds to take a couple of puffs before returning to their activity.

With asthma we can certainly offer every child complete freedom from the condition with a sensible logical assessment and treatment format as described in this book. No child should feel that their asthma is keeping them from enjoying life to the full and using this book will give you a treatment routine to suit your child.

If you follow this plan you should have a healthy child with treatment tailored to his or her individual situation. Hopefully you will never have to see your doctor except for repeat prescriptions of the relevant inhalers. Occasionally you may hit upon a doctor who does not fully grasp the complexities of the condition and may not treat your child vigorously enough. Do not accept second best but find a doctor who is more interested.

Equally you may have received sound advice but choose to ignore it because of something someone has said or perhaps a snippet of incorrect information on the television. By following the steps in this book you can be certain that the treatment will work, as it has been tried on many, many children. Please think twice before going off at a tangent, as you are taking a decision on behalf of your child which he or she has no power to understand. This book has been produced to lead you easily through the maze of treatments that are available so you will be confident of success whenever your child starts to wheeze.

We can be confident now that it is possible to control asthma and limit its effect so it plays little part in marring the quality of life. The perfect answer, however, would be to find a single cure that would rid the world of this condition and make the regular ingestion of different medications totally unnecessary. This is the real aim of the Asthma Research Council, and it is to be hoped that eventually a simple cure will be found.

The main problem in asthma is that the airways are very irritable so that certain stimuli can cause them to narrow. In children who do not suffer from it, their airways are not sensitive, so the same stimuli do not have any effect. Most research is aimed at finding the reason for this sensitivity, as if this can be established then a cure would be much nearer. It seems that there are two important factors and those are a genetic one and an environmental one. Genetic in its broadest sense means the family characteristics handed on from parents to children; undoubtedly if the parents have asthma it is much more likely – though by no means certain – that their children will develop it. The environmental influence includes the effects of cultural habits and lifestyle, or external factors such as climate or exposure to allergens.

It is interesting that almost half the inhabitants of the island of Tristan da Cunha have asthma and yet there are no extra provoking agents. The commonest allergen to be found there is the house-dust mite, just like in this country. It seems to be the inbreeding on Tristan da Cunha that is vital, as of the five original female inhabitants three had asthma, indicating that most of the asthma is handed down from generation to generation.

There is also no doubt that if you move children from a rural to an urban way of life then asthma increases dramatically. The most likely reasons are the increased pollution and faster, more stressful lifestyle in the towns and cities. However, it may be that it is something even more basic in that movement of people from the country to town is often associated with a decrease in the extent to which children are breast-fed. In the first six months of life the child's chief nourishment is from milk. If the mother's milk is replaced by cows' milk the exposure of the infant to foreign and potentially allergenic material will be increased. It has been shown that avoidance of cows' milk does reduce the chance of developing eczema which seems to have the same genetic and allergic basis as asthma. In Papua New Guinea asthma is virtually unknown and all children there are breast-fed. Whether this is in fact the sole reason for the freedom from breathing problems cannot be proved.

Apart from the question of breast-feeding there is a hypothesis that social differences are important. It was at one time suggested that children from upper social classes were more prone to asthma. This was put forward when school doctors' records in the Isle of Wight were analysed. Unfortunately a similar study amongst children in Aberdeen showed an excess of asthma in the children of semi-skilled and unskilled manual workers.

When you look at all the evidence, it appears certain that the dual influences of external and inherited forces are closely interlinked. Climatic and socio-economic circumstances cannot alone induce asthma to those not inherently predisposed. Equally, given an inherited tendency to asthma, the environment, whether this be in terms of exposure to allergens, adverse weather conditions, industrial pollution or domestic circumstances, can play a major role in actually triggering an attack.

Thus, whether viewed in the individual child or in whole communities, there is no escape from the conclusion that asthma is truly a multifactorial disorder and cannot be put down to a single cause. It is the summation of the effects of inheritance and environment that determines whether asthma will or will not be experienced. The addition of one further trigger factor, however minor it may be on its own, can be sufficient to bring the underlying tendency to asthma out into the open. If your child is fortunate not to combine enough of the trigger factors together at any one time, then the wheezing problem may never surface. Conversely what might itself be only a minor adjustment in environment or medical management may be all that is needed to convert a troublesome persistent asthma to a mild and occasional wheeze.

This complex situation explains why it is proving so difficult to find a single cure for asthma. Some day, no doubt, a remedy will be found but that time seems some way off. It is important to remember that while this cure does not yet exist, present-day treatment is very effective at both preventing the attacks developing and relieving any wheeze that may arise.

Why is it, then, that a number of children die from asthma every year if the treatment is so efficient? I am quite certain there are two main reasons: first, the therapy is not given in a logical fashion but in a rather haphazard irregular way. This may be the doctor's fault in not fully explaining the situation or it may be the parents' fault for not ensuring their child takes the recommended dosage. The second reason is that it has only recently been realized that while rapid narrowing of the airways by muscle spasm has always been assumed to be the main process in asthma, actual swelling of the airway linings is just as important and can come on much more insidiously. This is much slower to resolve and can lead to exhaustion. It is vital therefore if your child's peak flow is consistently below normal for you to see your doctor for assessment. The only really effective treatment for swelling of the linings is cortisone, either via an inhaler or in tablet form. If cortisone is used correctly in short sharp courses it is perfectly safe.

The introduction of asthma clinics has greatly improved the care of children with asthma as it means the parents have a place to go to discuss any problems that may arise. It also ensures they do not have to wait for an appointment but have open access to the doctor or nurse. Nor is there any reason to feel guilty about contacting your GP. For many parents it is a place to discuss their fears and worries, for example the question of taking cortisone. Hopefully in the next few years all surgeries will run these clinics so the standard of care will become much higher.

One of the most exciting developments in the past few years has been the increased interest and usage of alternative or complementary techniques in the management of asthma. Most of these are not given to cure the disease but to stimulate the vital force within the body to function efficiently. What we call disease is actually a decline of the vital force which drives the body's defences, and it is caused by anxiety, cold, eating too much, drinking too much, exhaustion, shock, inhaling polluted air, drink, food, liquids, fumes and so on. When the tone of the vital force within has been lowered, many things come out of balance, bacterial growth may find favourable conditions to increase, glands may produce too little or too much of their secretions; in fact a thousand things may go wrong, including the ability of the body to prevent the development of a wheezing attack.

The principle in acupuncture is to correct the obstruction of energy along the various channels in the body, thus restoring a normal flow of this energy or life force. Once this is done the body will then heal itself.

One of the main thrusts of homoeopathy - which is far more understandable now than in earlier times - is the use of minute doses. Hahnemann, the founder of homoeopathy taught that the smaller the potency of the drug administered the more easily it is absorbed by the sick body, which rejects strong doses. Remarkable cures have been recorded with this treatment since it was first instituted. Many medicines in several branches of healing are administered far too strongly. A sick body can make better use of smaller doses administered more frequently than it can of giant, powerful doses shoved down the gullet like a knock-out blow to a boxer. I know with conventional medicine that increasing the dose of medicine usually does not increase the chances of success in treatment but often just produces more unwanted effects.

When considering herbal medicine one of the fallacies advanced by allopaths is that herbs are too primitive, raw, impure and weak to be effective and that they are only usable when they have been concentrated, refined, turned into quintessential extracts and so on. This is absolutely untrue. As with other forms of alternative medicine, the herbalist is looking not specifically to cure the condition but to nourish the body and let it heal itself. It is ridiculous to suggest that they must do this in the same way as the conventional orthodox physicians do. If you take an old lady with hypothermia from the cold you do not warm her up very quickly, but gradually and gently. If someone is very dehydrated then it is vital to give them fluids slowly and with great care. So why should this be different with any other condition?

I believe we are entering upon an age of awareness when people all over the world are becoming conscious of a need for enlightenment and alive to the alternatives that are available. At present it is often necessary to take conventional medicine for asthma attacks as it is a serious condition. However, prevention of attacks is the real key to controlling the condition and alternative methods including acupuncture, homoeopathy, hypnosis and herbalism can all be used for this, and also be used where the wheezing is mild.

Through the passage of this book we have followed the progress of two children: Julie and Simon. I can still remember their initial attacks and all the worry and anxiety they caused. It was from their suffering and inspiration that this complete treatment plan arose. I know that it works as it is now some years since those traumatic days and I am glad to say that both Simon and Julie are growing up in a happy and healthy way, without restrictions on their lifestyle. So if you are unfortunate enough to have a child with asthma please do not despair. Take the time to read this book and follow the prevention and treatment plans. You can be certain then that your son or daughter will have a safe upbringing with minimal breathing problems. You owe it to your child to do just that.

I will close this book with an essay that Julie wrote at school and which her mother passed on to me. It should serve as an inspiration to all children with asthma and I have given it pride of place on my surgery noticeboard:

Last year I always seemed to be ill with my breathing and never seemed to be able to breathe properly like all my friends. Both my mum and dad were at work every day so they always asked my neighbour from next door to look after me. I didn't like her really as she had bad teeth and I wanted my mum. If it was weekend my big brother would stay with me but he played on the computer all the time and the noise drove me mad. One day I was given a syrup, but it was horrid and I threw it out of the window and it hit someone passing below. One day my mum took me to the doctors and I joined an asthma club. My number was 114 and instead of medicine I was given a little puffer which I squirted into my mouth to make my breathing better. The doctor let me borrow a special machine which I use when I am very wheezy. It is like being on a space ship as you have to wear a mask and breathe in this special cloud that comes out of the machine. The club is great and the nurse is very nice and always gives me a badge. We play a game where you have to blow as hard as you can into a little tube and see how far up the scale you can blow the pointer.

I have been to this club six times and now I hardly ever have any wheezing. Best of all when I am ill my mum stays with me until I am better. I love my mum, she is the best mum in the whole world.

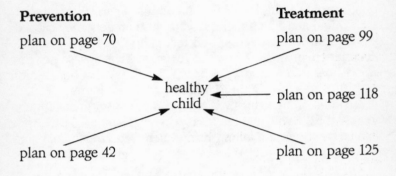

Prevention

plan on page 70

plan on page 42

healthy child

Treatment

plan on page 99

plan on page 118

plan on page 125

Complete treatment plan

Useful Addresses

UK

Associations

The Asthma Research Council
12 Pembridge Square, London W2 4EH

The Asthma Society
300 Upper Street, London N1 2XX (071-226 2260)

Asthma Swim Movement
45 Lickhill Road, Calne, Wilts SN11 9EZ

British Acupuncture Association
34 Alderney Street, London SW1V 4EU

British Homoeopathic Association
27a Devonshire Place, London W1N 1RJ (071-935 2163)

The Institute for Complementary Medicine
21 Portland Place, London W1N 3AF (071-636 9543)

National Council of Hypnotherapists
1 Clovelly Road, Ealing, London W5

National Society for Research into Allergy
PO Box 45, Hinckley, Leicester LE10 1JY (0455 635212)

Suppliers (Homoeopathic Medicine)

Ainsworths Homoeopathic Pharmacy
38 New Cavendish Street, London W1M 7LH (071-935 5330)
40-44 High Street, Caterham, Surrey CR3 5UB (0883 40332)

Freemans Homoeopathic Pharmacy
7 Eaglesham Road, Glasgow G76 7BU (041-644 4640)

Nelsons Homoeopathic Pharmacy
73 Duke Street, London W1M 6BY (071-629 3118)

Weleda (UK) Ltd
Heanor Road, Ilkeston, Derby DE7 8DR (0602 303151)

Winchester Homoeopathic Dispensary
11 Bridge Street, Winchester, Hampshire SO23 8HL
(0962 53260)

Australia

Associations

Australian Asthma Foundation
82-86 Pacific Highway, St Leonards, 2065 NSW (02 906 3233)
2 Highfield Grove, Kew, 3102 VIC (03 861 5666)
PO Box 394, Fortitude Valley, 4006 QLD (07 252 7677)
341 Halifax Street, Adelaide, 5000 SA (08 223 7235)
2/61 Heytesbury Road, Subiaco, 6008 WA (09 382 1666)
PO Box 40456, Casuarina, Darwin, 0811 NT (089 208817)
82 Hampden Road, Battery Point, 7000 TAS (002 237725)

Index